the ten hidden barriers to
WEIGHT LOSS & EXERCISE

**discover why
you've failed
before & how to
succeed now**

LYNETTE A. MENEFEE, PH.D.
DANIEL R. SOMBERG, PH.D.

New Harbinger Publications, Inc.

Publisher's Note

This publication is designed to provide accurate and authoritative information in regard to the subject matter covered. It is sold with the understanding that the publisher is not engaged in rendering psychological, financial, legal, or other professional services. If expert assistance or counseling is needed, the services of a competent professional should be sought.

Distributed in the U.S.A. by Publishers Group West; in Canada by Raincoast Books; in Great Britain by Hi Marketing, Ltd.; in South Africa by Real Books, Ltd.; in Australia by Boobook; and in New Zealand by Tandem Press.

Copyright © 2003 by Lynette A. Menefee and Daniel R. Somberg
New Harbinger Publications, Inc.
5674 Shattuck Avenue
Oakland, CA 94609

Cover design by Amy Shoup
Text design by Tracy Marie Carlson

ISBN 1-57224-324-4 Paperback

New Harbinger Publications' Web site address: www.newharbinger.com

05   04   03

10   9   8   7   6   5   4   3   2   1

First printing

To my sister, Laurie Jane
—L. M.

To my wife, Kelly
—D. S.

Contents

Acknowledgments

I would like to thank my sister, Laurie, for her wise counsel and for listening with a discerning ear and a tender heart. Only she could know me well enough to write out my goals for the year, albeit on a styrofoam cup. I would like to thank God for blessing me with other encouraging family members: my parents, Lynn and Helen; and my brothers and their wives, Bruce and Ruth and Paul and Nickie; and their children, Joshua, Madeline, and Evan, who bring me joy. I thank special friends; among them Jerry Fuller, and Kim Sanschagrin, two people who encouraged me to write and listened during the process. Finally, I would like to note that the order of authorship in this book was determined by a coin toss that I still believe my coauthor should have won.
—L. M.

I would like to thank my parents and my brother and sister—Suzanne, Ray, Ken, and Debra—for their love and unwavering confidence in me. I also want to thank all my other family members and friends for their enthusiasm and support throughout this project. I am very grateful to Bruce Liese for the generous sharing of his clinical experience and wisdom. I thank my children, Zach and Lindsay, for their love, excitement, and patience during this process, and for just being such wonderful kids. And finally, I want to thank my wife Kelly for her love, support, and dedication to our family, which allowed me to complete this book and helps me to stay on track with what is most important in life.

—D. S.

We would also like to thank Heather Mitchener and Tesilya Hanauer at New Harbinger Publications for their wonderful input and direction throughout the writing of this book.

And lastly, thanks to all of our patients who have taught us about the challenges and obstacles in pursuing their goals, and the courage needed to face them directly.

—L. M. and D. S.

Introduction

Many Americans are trying to shed unwanted and unhealthy excess weight, as a thirty-three-billion-dollar weight-loss industry can attest. A quick look in the bookstore will remind you that there is no shortage of prescriptive, "do this, don't do that" plans for weight loss and exercise. Some are based on a solid foundation of well-studied methods, while others are based on myths and fads, both old and new. Unfortunately, research studies have repeatedly shown that most dieters have similar results, regardless of the method they choose: an initial weight loss, followed by an eventual return to baseline weight.

We aren't going to offer you yet another weight-loss plan, and we won't be describing new exercise techniques either. That's because for many people, the path to success is straightforward: you need to understand and change the key behaviors and thought patterns that relate to successful weight loss and exercise. This book will describe these and show you how to apply them to your own life. We will assume your knowledge, past experience, and common sense tell you a good deal about what a sensible weight-loss and exercise plan looks like. While we will briefly review some of the more tried-and-true basics of what you should do in your weight-loss and exercise plan, the primary focus of this book is to teach you how to identify and overcome hidden barriers that keep you from success.

Your Challenge: Staying on Track

Making the decision to exercise regularly and eat healthy foods often leads to a frustrating cycle of good intentions and not-so-good follow-through. Odds are that you could do a reasonably good job of telling a friend or neighbor what they should do to lose weight and exercise regularly. Unfortunately, telling someone else what to do is infinitely easier than guiding yourself. (Maybe this is why being told what you should do by others is often unappreciated and a bit irritating.) Why is this so? Changes you want to make must happen within the context of your many other priorities and influences, such as pangs of hunger, desire for comfort, unpleasant emotions, expectations of others, and home and work responsibilities. Once you add in a lifetime of past learning and experiences, it becomes clear that losing weight and exercising are far from the only things on your plate. Our goal is to help you understand what to do and how to guide yourself in doing it, *within the context of your unique life.*

How do you make sense of why you weren't able to change habits successfully in the past? You might be inclined to chalk it up to laziness, tiredness, or just being too busy. Unfortunately, these explanations are overly simplistic and often derogatory. Besides that, they don't offer much guidance about what you might do differently. Depending on your style, maybe you just skip any kind of explanation and go right to being angry or simply giving up. It's as if you have some hidden barrier that prevents you from reaching your goals—if only you could find it. This book aims to help you find accurate explanations for your past difficulties and to teach you the basics of habit change that are so essential to weight loss and exercise.

With each chapter, you will find insights and strategies to identify your particular reasons for getting off track from your plan, and you will be guided to understand why and how this happens. You'll find out about various reasons you end up getting off track, including not believing you can really do it, impulsively responding to uncomfortable emotions, reacting to your mistakes in a harsh manner, or finding your attention and energy being directed toward meeting others' expectations. By identifying the barriers that cause you to get off track and looking at them in a nonjudgmental way, you will be in a position to address the issue directly and effectively, rather than letting it hide safely buried beneath your frustration and repeated disappointments.

Turning Barriers into Solutions

Managing a project, any project, toward successful completion requires a person to do a number of things well. You must know what needs to be done, motivate yourself to do it, keep your focus on your goal, manage distractions, and maintain morale, among other factors. This book describes ten similar skills and resources that will help you achieve your weight loss and exercise goals. A barrier occurs when you are having difficulty with one of these ten areas and it is causing you to get off track. While you may be very aware of not reaching your healthy goals, your particular barriers to success often remain "hidden."

Each barrier highlights an important ingredient needed for successful change. Difficulty in each area can be frustrating, especially if it is not identified or well understood. We encourage you to think of each barrier as an opportunity to understand, learn, confront, and overcome. We know it can be done, and we'll offer you advice about how to do it.

Using This Book

You may want to use this book to get a comprehensive understanding of the many important components to making lasting change. The strategies offered here will help you practice and incorporate the solutions into your game plan. We also recommend using this book to help you identify your particular challenges and difficulties. Once the difficulty is identified, you may find you already have the resources to focus on and resolve the problem. However, you may also need to use the book to identify the problem and then go on to get more in-depth attention and assistance to address the issue.

One final note: We encourage you to read this book with a sense of optimism and hope. It may not come easily, so you may have to fake it at first. Why? First, it's just a good idea. A positive outlook and expectation are very helpful in creating change. Second, you have good reason to be optimistic. You have taken on challenges before and accomplished them. And when you haven't been able to accomplish your goals, there was a reason. Now, you will be armed with a better understanding of what is getting you off track and with more tools and strategies than ever before.

Are You Ready for Change?

If you're like most people, there are many things that you wish could be different in your life. You may want to lose weight, stop smoking, be more assertive, learn another language, or spend more time with a loved one. Some of the things you will do, others you won't. So what determines whether you achieve your goals? A very important factor in determining this answer is your readiness to change. If not sufficiently developed, your level of readiness can be a barrier to reaching your weight loss and exercise goals. This chapter will help you understand and identify your current readiness to change your habits and provide strategies for increasing your readiness.

What Is Readiness to Change?

Much of the scientific research about making healthy lifestyle changes—such as losing weight, exercising, quitting smoking, and reducing alcohol consumption—has focused on the degree to which people are really ready for change. The results show that real change occurs only when a person is ready. The good news is that at some level you *are* ready, because you're reading this book and trying to understand why your attempts thus far haven't been as successful as you would like. In this chapter, you will learn how ambivalence, or simultaneous thoughts of wanting and not wanting something, keeps you from being fully ready to change.

Why would you be ambivalent about a potentially positive change? Actually, there are several possible explanations. For example, how important is changing to you? If the desire to change is more important to someone else (your spouse, family, or doctor) than it is to you, this can contribute to ambivalence about changing. Another factor is the degree of confidence you have that you can make the changes you want. If you don't really think that you can lose weight or maintain an exercise program, or you believe that nothing will help, then you'll be ambivalent about trying to change. How do the advantages of making the change compare to the advantages of staying the same? How do you view the disadvantages of trying to change? Your answers to these questions help determine your readiness to change. You have reasons to change and reasons to stay the same and you need to be aware of both to resolve ambivalence and move ahead toward your goal.

A Readiness to Change Model

The question you may be asking yourself is, "How can I change for good?" One possible answer to this question comes from a well-researched theory proposed by psychologists Prochaska and DiClemente (1983). These scientists suggest that readiness to change occurs in predictable stages that advance from not thinking about change to contemplating, enacting, and maintaining change. A person can go back and forth between the stages of readiness and wind up at the beginning after a lapse. Below are some descriptions of the stages of change.

Precontemplation Stage

The precontemplation stage is the first stage of change—the one in which you are not considering changing at all. Some people are in a state of denial that there will be any adverse consequences of their health habits. Even if they acknowledge that there may be some problems, they minimize the extent of the problems or think that bad effects won't happen to them. Individuals in the precontemplation stage may point to others who have averted negative health consequences for their behaviors, blame others for their problems, or express happiness with the way things are. They may say, "I've tried exercising regularly before and it doesn't work," or "Nothing works for me, so I might as well accept that this is how I am."

Contemplation Stage

You might guess that the next stage of change, called contemplation, involves beginning to think about change. In the contemplation stage, you begin to be aware of your state as opposed to other, possibly more desirable states. In this stage, you are more aware of the reasons you want to change and you may begin to think about seeking information regarding exercise and a healthy diet.

Preparation Stage

The next stage of change is called preparation. If you are in the preparation stage, you are generally preparing to make changes within the next month. Have you thought about what you will do to achieve your weight-loss and exercise goals? Do you know about exercise offerings in your area? Do you have a weight-loss goal? Even though you may be planning for action, your ambivalence may still be high. If you skip this stage, or rush through it without making concrete plans, you may be short-circuiting your chances for long-term success.

Action Stage

The action stage is next. In this stage, your actions are visible and can be observed by others. Someone following you around with a video camera would easily record the actions you take toward reaching your goal. This is a busy stage, the one in which you may begin to feel some satisfaction that you have started making changes.

Most organized weight-loss and exercise programs, books, and magazine articles encourage you to "just do it." But Prochaska's research has shown that only 20 percent of people are ready for an action approach at any given time. Therefore, a premature move to action is a mistake that actually does a disservice to your long-term progress. It is vitally important that you move toward action at your own pace and that you work within your stage of change until you are truly ready to move toward action. Only then will action be sustained for the long haul.

Maintenance Stage

The maintenance stage is the stage in which you maintain the action toward your goal. This stage is a little like brushing your teeth every night. The behavior becomes a habit that is maintained over time. Many people make it to the action stage in adopting a new health behavior at one time or another. You have probably tried losing weight and increasing exercise before. If so, you know that maintaining the initial gains can be a difficult process. The two major dangers in the maintenance phase are: overconfidence that permanent change has occurred, and not planning for lapses that could turn into relapses that send you back to the earliest stages of change.

Termination Stage

Most people cycle through the stages of change several times before their behavior patterns become so permanent that they can confidently say that they'll never have trouble with the behavior again. Some problems don't have a termination stage; instead, there comes a time when the problem becomes less salient because you have the skills to handle slips and temptations. You'll know you're in the termination stage when a new self-image is developed and there is no temptation to return to the old behavior. Additionally, you will have developed many strategies that work for you when you are in tempting situations, and you'll have confidence that you can use these strategies well.

How Quickly Can Change Happen?

Professionals working with individuals to help them change their eating and exercising behaviors sometimes encounter a person who appears to move from the precontemplation stage to the action and maintenance stages almost immediately. In this situation, the person changes dramatically and for good. Why? First, individuals who appear to change rapidly are probably among the 20 percent of people who are truly ready for action. They have likely gone through the stages, just much more quickly than most people do. Sometimes this type of change occurs after a traumatic life experience, a personal awakening, or a sudden insight. Think of it as a permanent "ah-ha" that leads to action and long-term change. Some individuals who have lost weight and kept it off for many years describe an event (or series of events) that was their personal turning point.

Some people are motivated by a crisis or a personal awakening that shakes them from the status quo and moves them to act in their own best interest. Although dramatic change happens at times and is the kind of change highlighted in the media, the vast majority of change is made after deliberate contemplation and consideration of the same topics presented in this book. In the next section, you will learn more about your particular stage of change and how you can facilitate your readiness.

Knowing your level of readiness to lose weight and maintain an exercise program is extremely important. Many people expect themselves to jump into action before they have fully thought through what the consequences of the action might be. Without preparing for change, a thirty-year, three-pack-per-day cigarette smoker is unlikely to quit cold turkey and never return to smoking. This person must first understand more about the challenges of stopping smoking and then construct a viable plan for what to do when the urge to smoke hits or when a friend who smokes offers a cigarette after dinner. Although jumping to action sometimes brings about results in the short term, most of the time you simply set yourself up for failure if you expect action without preparation. With preparation, the long-term results are more likely to be positive.

In this book, no presumption is made that now is the best time for you to change, nor is it assumed that you want to confront any ambivalence you may have. Maybe you will choose to move slightly, but not fully, toward action. Perhaps you will make a decision not to change at all. The goal of this chapter is to help you learn whether your readiness level has been stopping you from achieving your goal. If it has, and you want to move toward actions you can maintain over time, we will happily show you how. Otherwise, you can use what you learn here to acknowledge that you aren't quite ready to change in the ways you thought. You can stop blaming yourself for not having what it takes to succeed, and you'll know where to start to increase your success when you are ready.

How Are You Doing Now?

Complete the following exercises for some clues about whether your readiness to change is keeping you from moving toward your goals. Read the following statements and check off the ones that describe you most closely.

☐ I read about how to make changes, but don't do it myself.

☐ I have made changes in the past, but then go back to my old habits.

☐ My behaviors may cause future problems, but it's hard for me to do anything about them.

☐ Thinking about what it would take to change is overwhelming.

☐ I know my own reasons for seeking to change right now.

☐ I am taking actions to reach my goals.

☐ I am confident in my ability to permanently change my habits.

☐ I have solved most of my problems related to changing my lifestyle.

If the first four statements describe you best, then some of the reasons you may not be as successful as you would like may be related to your readiness for change. If the last four statements describe you best, then you may be on your way. Regardless, you are still encouraged to read this chapter and do the exercises to help reinforce and understand where you are.

Determine Your Stage of Change

Prochaska and colleagues have an easy way to determine your stage of change. For the purposes of defining your stage of change, and in defining what it means to "take action" in the assessment below we will use a somewhat arbitrary goal. (In the next chapter, we will help you refine your goal.) For now, if your goal is to lose weight, count yourself as having taken action if you are losing one to two pounds per week toward a healthy weight. If your goal is to increase exercise, count yourself as having taken action if you are exercising at a moderate pace for at least twenty minutes five times per week. Again, these are arbitrary goals, but they'll provide a marker for defining your stage of change.

Your stage of change for weight loss and exercise will likely be different, so think about each area in the the following terms. If you can say that you solved your difficulties with weight loss (or exercise) at least six months ago, you are in the maintenance stage. If you took action within the last six months, but have not solved your weight-loss (or exercise) problems, you are in the action stage. Do you plan to take action on your weight-loss (or exercise) goals within the next month to six months? Then you are in the preparation stage. If you are thinking about taking action on your weight-loss (or exercise) goals within the next six months, you are in the contemplation stage. Finally, if you are not intending to take action on your weight-loss (or exercise) goals at this time, you are in the precontemplation stage. Now that you know your initial stages, let's explore your readiness for change in more depth.

How Can You Be More Successful?

To be more successful, you can advance your readiness to change. Although the exercises presented below are generally most appropriate for the earlier stages of change, you are encouraged to think carefully about the exercises in each section, since the cycle of change may be experienced several times before more permanent change occurs.

Balance the Pros and Cons

You've no doubt used a pro and con list to think about a problem before. Behavioral scientists have found that individuals often do not investigate the pros and cons of *both* sides of a behavior. This tool will help you learn more about what motivates you to lose weight and exercise. One important aspect of this tool is being honest with yourself about the positive aspects of what you are doing now. You receive some rewards for doing what you are doing now or you wouldn't be doing it.

Take a sheet of paper and draw a line down the middle. Then draw a horizonal line midway down the page. First, concentrate on weight loss. Write the word "pros" above the left-hand boxes and the word "cons" above the right-hand side. On the "pro" side, write the following in the top box: "What are the benefits of my current eating habits?" and this in the bottom box: "What are the benefits of losing weight?" On the "con" side, write the following in the top box: "What concerns me about not losing weight?" and this in the bottom box: "What concerns me about losing weight?" Take a few minutes to focus on each block and answer each question to the best of your knowledge.

Now turn the paper over and answer the same questions related to exercise. On the "pro" side, answer: "What are the benefits of not exercising?" and "What are the benefits of exercising?" On the "con" side, answer: "What concerns me about not exercising?" and "What concerns me about exercising?" Take a few minutes to focus on each question and answer as honestly as you can.

When you complete the exercise, you will have listed both the reasons you would like to change and the reasons you would like to stay as you are. There is important information that you can learn from this exercise to help you move up a stage in the stages of change. However, the main purpose of this exercise is to explore your thoughts; it's not intended to change your mind about what to do. Remember that what you ultimately decide about moving to the action and maintenance stages is entirely up to you. Complete the following to get the most out of listing the pros and cons.

Sum It Up

To see the big picture, look over the pros and cons of changing and of staying the same. Take out a sheet of paper and sum it up in one paragraph, making an executive summary of your situation. Your summary gives you a succinct overall picture of some of your thoughts about changing. Prochaska and colleagues (1994) show that there is a pattern of pros and cons that facilitates movement from stage to stage. In the initial stages (precontemplation to contemplation), concentrate on increasing the pros of losing weight and exercising. In later stages (contemplation to action), concentrate on decreasing the cons, or the problems you perceive with losing weight and exercising. As the benefits of changing your habits become more apparent, you are more likely to actually change.

Keep in mind that moving ahead is not as simple as listing the pros and cons. The importance of one pro or con on either side may outweigh all of the others. Find the most important reason for staying the same and the most important reason for changing and complete this sentence: "On one hand, I (*insert best reason for staying the same*), but on the other hand (*insert your best reason for changing*)." Simply writing out this statement is helpful in seeing the "bottom line" of your behaviors. Now, rate the strength of those reasons on a scale of 0 (not important at all) to 100 (extremely important). After isolating and rating the most important benefit and challenge, you can explore the ambivalence that is normal when you begin to think about changing.

Find the Right Information

Exploring ambivalence involves obtaining the right information. Sometimes what keeps you from moving forward are beliefs that are based on inaccuracies. In the early stages of change, look at the pros and cons to uncover excuses that may not be based on fact. Some common reasons people give for not changing are: "It takes too much time," "It takes too much energy," "I've tried before and nothing works," "Someone else has control because they buy or prepare the food in the house," "I don't have money," and "I wouldn't know who I was if I changed."

Start asking some questions about whether these beliefs are accurate. Finding the right information may mean talking with a doctor, nurse, or registered dietitian. It may mean discussing the situation with your family members or friends. Tell them your situation and ask them whether they think your beliefs are true and if they can offer other suggestions. Try turning the statements around, such as by asking, "What is the least amount of time/energy/money that it would take for me to begin to lose weight and exercise?" Your beliefs may be realistic. Family finances may not allow you to join a gym or participate in a YMCA. However, there *are* many low- and no-cost ways to exercise that will increase your endurance and improve your health. Open your mind to exploring both sides of your ambivalence and collect important information that you can factor into the pro and con balance sheet.

Look Ahead

Another technique for moving through your current stage of change is to project yourself into the future and see what the continuation of your behaviors will bring. Ask yourself, "What would it be like if I didn't change my behavior?" What would be happening in your life? What would be likely to happen next? How would you feel?

Project into the future again, this time envisioning what life might be like if you obtained your goals. Imagine your feelings about yourself and potential reactions from others. Some people are motivated by images that bring home the risk of not changing while others are motivated by visualizing the positive possibilities in the future. The point of this exercise is to help you connect with the emotions related to the changes you want to make. This technique may help motivate you toward action, and can be used to reinforce your change when you feel tempted in the action and maintenance stages. This exercise only takes a minute. So, close your eyes right now and imagine your life, together with the thoughts, feelings, surroundings, and reactions from others that might occur in both future scenarios. Now, ask yourself what you will have to do now to make the future what you want it to be.

Check Your Values and Beliefs

Your values and beliefs are important for change. Your values, or what's most important to you, guide what you do each day. As you think about your daily activities, rate the importance of losing weight, eating healthy foods, and exercising separately on three scales that range from 0 (not important at all) to 100 (very important). You should have a value rating for weight loss, a value rating for eating healthy foods, and a value rating for exercise. If your value rating for each of these lifestyle behaviors is high, then they should be reflected in your daily life. Ask yourself if these values are represented at the level you would like them to be. What do you need to do to increase your ratings?

Now, rate the belief you have that you can accomplish your goals with respect to weight loss and exercise. Use the 0 (no confidence) to 100 (absolute confidence) scale to rate your confidence in the following statements: 1) I believe in my ability to lose weight, 2) I know I can reach my exercise goal, and 3) I choose to eat more healthy foods.

How high are your ratings? If you have difficulties believing that you have what it takes to accomplish your goals, then increasing your confidence will help you get ready for action. Ask yourself what you would have to do to increase your confidence rating by 10 points. One way to increase your confidence is to create a positive experience. Here's how it works: simply think about the confidence you had the last time you reached a weight loss or exercise milestone. But there's more. Practicing the recommendations presented in this book will provide you with many additional positive experiences, showing you that you *can* indeed reach your goals. Choose an easy action to perform today, such as having a serving of vegetables with a meal or as a snack. Another way to increase your confidence is to watch someone else succeed, paying attention when they make healthy choices. Consider implementing one of their healthy choices or another new strategy you've heard about.

Develop Empathy

You can help yourself through the early stages of change, when you are most ambivalent, by developing empathy toward yourself and others. Developing empathy toward yourself involves adopting an attitude of understanding and acceptance that you are moving forward, even if it seems like the movement is at a snail's pace.

In addition to trying to facilitate this attitude toward yourself, try to understand how others feel about your current habits and/or the changes you want to make. Put yourself in their position and attempt to understand what they are trying to tell you. What you perceive as nagging might just be a concern that they have for their own security if your health is endangered. What you perceive as negative comments that are unhelpful may be the only way they know of attempting to motivate you. Developing empathy with yourself and others early in the process will help you progress through the stages of change.

Later Stage Exercises

Tasks that take place in the preparation, action, and maintenance stages involve planning, committing, and taking action. Solutions you can use in the preparation stage are covered in the next chapter where we help you be more specific about the goals you are trying to reach and outline a successful game plan. Solutions for beginning to take action and maintaining gains are presented in later chapters as well.

Why Are You Getting off Track?

What happens if you have trouble being truly ready to change? Check to see if any of the following might be increasing the likelihood that you are getting off track.

- Are you engaging in wishful thinking that weight loss and exercise will happen by themselves, or at least very quickly?

- Are you unclear about what is motivating you?

- Have you jumped to action too soon, without being prepared for the change?

- Do you value your health enough that a healthy lifestyle is a daily priority?

- Do you feel ambivalence when you think about weight loss and exercise?

Strategies for Staying on Track

The following strategies can help you stay on track when you feel your readiness to change waning.

Redo the Pros and Cons Balance Sheet

If you get off track, redo the pros and cons balance sheet for more information about your thinking about change. This exercise will help you be honest about your motivations for change.

Make the Future Real

Realistically look at all of the effects you will expect if you continue with your present patterns. If you need to, go out and get information about what will happen if you maintain your current unhealthy habits.

Allow Time to Prepare for Change

To avoid jumping to action before you are ready, make it your short-term goal to contemplate the changes and prepare for them.

Read Chapter 2

If you are having trouble placing a high daily value on your health, read the next chapter for some clues about defining your priorities and your lifestyle goals.

Are Your Goal and Game Plan Right for You?

Creating good goals and a workable game plan is a critical part of helping you stay on track with your healthy goals. An inappropriate goal or poorly developed game plan can be a barrier to carrying out your wonderful intentions to change. In this chapter, you'll learn to make good goals, ones that you can sustain with a reasonable amount of effort. You will also create and evaluate your game plan for achieving these goals. Along the way, we'll review a few basics of health information so you can ensure that your goals are on track. The purpose of this chapter is to help you put your goals to an acid test and double-check your game plan to see if it's truly right for you.

What Is Your Goal?

Most people can define a goal. A goal is an endpoint toward which we direct our efforts. It is rare, however, to find an individual who can distinguish a well-constructed goal that is likely to be accomplished from an ill-conceived goal that there is little hope of attaining. Defining good weight loss and exercise goals can be tricky.

Goals have several distant cousins for which they are regularly mistaken. These are wishes, wants, and needs. Wishes are more fantasy than reality, and generally consist of something that is currently unattainable or unlikely to happen. Common wishes are for more hours in the day, instantaneous wealth, or perhaps a reversal of a negative event. Think about something for which you might wish. You might wish that you had the physique of a bathing suit model, could marry a movie star, or would win the lottery. But alas, only a small minority (think a teeny, tiny, minuscule number) of individuals on the planet will experience these things.

A want involves more desire than a wish and is more realistic and possible to attain. That's because wanting something enough may entice you to reprioritize your values and goals. You may have some wants that are unattainable, but you are more likely to exert effort for something you want. However, such a reorganization of values isn't certain, because wants can still be abstract or not translated into action. For example, you may want to exercise three times a week, but regular exercise may never make your active goal list.

The only thing that beats wishes and wants hands down is true need. What you want is one thing; what you truly need is another. But be careful. Wants and wishes can be stated as "needs," as in when you say, "I need to exercise today" when you know you are just wishing that you would exercise. Think about what you really, truly need in life. Your list of needs is bound to be more substantial and important to your core being than wishes and wants. When you satisfy a need, you fulfill a deeper purpose. When you have a real need to feel healthy, you naturally make it an important part of your everyday life. The value of healthy lifestyle behaviors will rise and your actions will follow. Now, let's revisit the definition of a goal. Goals guide actions that are directed toward meeting an end, preferably a true need to be and feel healthier. Meeting your true need through achieving lifestyle goals will lead to feelings of contentment and fulfillment.

What Is Your Game Plan?

A game plan is a strategy, or a set of strategies, to achieve an objective. In sports, a game plan is carefully devised to capitalize on the strengths of one team over the other. The coach designs plays that the team will be able to execute and that have a likelihood for success. A game plan is a step-by-step plan designed to meet the goal of winning the game. For example, if your goal is to increase the amount of exercise you do, then a beginning plan might be to find a type of exercise you like. A second step might be to learn where you can perform the exercise on a regular basis. A third step might be to plan a schedule that slowly begins to include exercise. A game plan for choosing healthy foods will include strategies of how to handle situations in which you are tempted to overeat.

A good game plan is important because each day you are faced with many choices related to your lifestyle goals. You'll use the specific strategies in your game plan to make these choices in a way that is consistent with your overall goals. These strategies will provide focus and incentive to keep you moving toward your goal, making your progress visible and sustainable. Evaluating your game plan to be sure that the daily actions you choose are related to your goal and are specific and reasonable is critical to meeting your overall goal. Without a workable game plan, it's unlikely you'll reach your goals.

Many, many people veer off track completely because they don't follow the rules for making good goals and implementing a game plan. Without knowing and following these rules, you can easily get stuck in a cycle of failure and frustration. The following exercises will help you think through your goals and your game plan so that you'll have confidence that you know where you're going, and you won't wind up somewhere else.

How Are You Doing Now?

Read the statements below and check off the ones that describe you best.

☐ I have defined priorities related to my health.

☐ I know where health ranks with my other life priorities.

☐ I have several specific, long-term goals related to my health.

☐ My goals are easily translated into my daily activities.

☐ I know when I have accomplished my goals.

☐ It is easy to see how my daily choices help me meet my health goals.

If you answered "yes" to the majority of these questions, then you are probably on the right track. If you answered "no" to a majority of these questions, then you may have more to learn about setting goals and creating a game plan. Whether you are on the right track or not, read on for suggestions on how to make your goals the best they can be to serve your purposes.

How Can You Be More Successful?

The following exercises will help you set good goals and create a game plan that will work for you. The process will require some thinking and figuring, so find a notebook or pad of paper before you begin.

Start with the Endpoint

Take a minute to review your healthy lifestyle goals. Is your overall goal to lose weight or adopt a regular exercise program? Do you want to meet a specific health objective, such as lowering your blood pressure? What lifestyle goals would meet your true need? If you met your healthy lifestyle goals, what would your life look like?

Write down the top four health-related goals (endpoints) you would like to achieve. By the end of this chapter, you will have put your goals to an acid test for soundness. First, we'll explain a few rules of good goals. Then, you'll use these rules to learn in more depth whether your goals are the best ones for you. Let's start by looking at four rules for good goals:

Good Goals Fit in with Your Overall Life Plan

Your goals for any one segment of your life, such as your family, your career, or your finances, are only as good as their fit into the overall plan for your life. You have an overall life plan, even if you don't know it. As discussed in the last chapter, your daily actions are a statement of your beliefs, your values, and what's important to you. Your general ideas about how to improve your health are among those beliefs and values.

It's easy to neglect weight loss and exercise goals when you haven't experienced negative consequences of poor health habits. On the other hand, overfocusing on health goals can keep you from being fully engaged in other, more important aspects of life.

Good Goals Are Reasonable and Sustainable

This rule for goals sounds so obvious that you might think it doesn't need to be stated. Not so! Most people who want to lose weight and increase exercise create goals that are unrealistic. Have you ever decided to exercise after a long sedentary period and said, "Starting today, I'm going to run a mile every day"? How about, "My goal is to lose fifteen pounds in a month"? Are these goals reasonable? Probably not.

Good Goals Are Well-Stated

Goals need to be stated in a positive and specific manner. If you said, "I will try to exercise for thirty minutes per day," would you be motivated? A more positive step forward is to say, "I will take a brisk walk on Monday, Wednesday, and Friday for thirty minutes. On Tuesday, Thursday and Saturday I will swim at the gym for forty-five minutes. Sunday, I will rest." Should you make this goal if you haven't exercised in years? You'd be right if you said, "No!" This goal sounds more like a long-term goal than a beginning goal. You'll need to write your goals in positive language that is specific to your situation.

Good Goals Are Measurable

Good goals are measurable, which means that it is possible to see if you have met them. A goal such as, "I will do something to improve my health," is too general to be measurable. A goal to maintain your current weight over the next two weeks is measurable by the scale. A goal to eat 1500 calories per day is measurable. After you establish your goals, you'll ask yourself how you will know that you accomplished your goal. Can you measure it? How will you measure it?

Take a Close Look

Your overall goals must fit in with your life plan, as discussed in the first rule of good goals. Use your notebook to list the top priorities in your life. Now, rank the importance of each of your priorities. Ranking the priorities is extremely important because the actions you perform each day should be determined by these priorities. Next, write down the answers to the following questions:

1. Where do your weight loss and exercise goals fit into your list of life priorities?

2. Is the ranking high enough that you act on it?

3. Are your lifestyle goals overshadowing more important priorities?

4. Would your priorities change if you began to suffer adverse health consequences?

5. What would it take for you to commit to making health a priority in your life plan?

Be Sure Your Goals Are Reasonable

Because setting reasonable goals is such an important part of staying on track, the following section will provide some basic weight-loss and exercise information to help you determine whether your goals are reasonable for you. This is the only time in the book that specific health information will be presented. The information provided here comes from *The Dietary Guidelines for Americans 2000* and can be found on the Internet (see Resources). The information presented is a general guideline, so we encourage you to talk with your physician about what is right for you. A registered dietitian may also be helpful.

The following sections will help you answer critical questions about the reasonableness of your weight loss and exercise goals. First, you will answer the following questions: Do you need to lose weight? If so, how much do you need to lose?

Find Your BMI

To find out whether you need to lose weight, you need to evaluate your weight in relation to your height. This results in something called Body Mass Index, or BMI. You will need to know your weight and height. The formula for BMI is:

[Weight in pounds/Height in inches/Height in inches] x 703

If you were 200 pounds and six feet tall, your BMI would be 200 pounds divided by seventy-two inches divided by seventy-two inches, multiplied by 703. You can also use an online BMI calculator (see Resources). Use these benchmarks for healthy weight:

- Healthy Weight = BMI from 18.5 to 24.9

- Overweight = BMI from 25 to 29.9

- Obese = BMI of 30 or higher.

If you have lots of muscle and little fat, then your BMI may be high, but your health risks will be lower than that BMI might otherwise indicate.

Consider Other Factors

Even if your BMI is in the healthy range, other factors may increase your risks for health problems. One of these factors is excess abdominal fat. Other factors include a family history of health problems, such as diabetes, heart disease, or high cholesterol. More information on other factors that make losing weight important can be found online (see Resources).

Decide How Much Weight You Need to Lose

Ideally, you will decide how much weight you need to lose with a physician and perhaps with the help of a registered dietitian. The task could look daunting if you have a BMI of thirty or higher. The good news is that new studies show that small amounts of weight loss (between 5 and 15 percent of your body weight) can delay or prevent diseases like diabetes (Knowler et al, 2002) and improve health (*Dietary Guidelines for Americans* 2000). A first step might be to lose weight within this range. Even though your BMI may not be in the healthy range after losing this percentage, you will still decrease the chances of illnesses associated with obesity.

Understand Which Methods Work Best

There are many ways to lose weight, as you are no doubt aware. Ask your doctor for an opinion about what may be right for you. In general, the Dietary Guidelines recommend that you lose weight the old-fashioned way—by doing so slowly and by changing your eating and exercise habits. If your BMI is in the obese range, you may want to consult a specialist to determine whether a special weight-loss program, medication, or surgery is right for you. You will still need to learn how to change your eating and exercise habits, but these alone may not be enough to help you meet your goals.

Lose Weight Slowly

A reasonable goal for most people is about 10 percent of their body weight over six months. This usually averages out to between a half-pound and two pounds per week. After you find a reasonable goal, you can figure out a schedule that works for you. Goals must be incremental, beginning a little at a time. If your BMI is high, a weight loss of 10 percent can be a starting goal that you will revise when you reach it. Multiply your current weight by .10 to find 10 percent of your body weight. If you're the hypothetical 200-pound person we mentioned earlier, that would be twenty pounds. Now, figure that a safe bet is to lose approximately one pound per week. It will take about twenty weeks (five months) to lose the desired weight.

What if you have eighty pounds to lose to move your BMI into a healthy range? Don't be discouraged. Remember that your goal is for weight loss you can sustain for a long time. In the race between the tortoise and the hare, the tortoise won. The consequences of being the hare, that is, finding a quick-fix crash diet, will ultimately put you further behind in the race. Think of the benefits of the goal described above. First, losing 10 percent of your body weight and keeping it off will help you feel better and will decrease some of the health risks associated with being overweight. Second, you will have learned lifestyle behaviors that will become habit, and the next milestone won't seem as hard to reach.

Eat Healthy Foods and Exercise

A healthy diet and exercise are recommended for long-term weight loss. Exercise will be discussed in the next section and is very important for overall health and for losing weight and maintaining weight loss. There are many good resources that describe how to eat more healthy foods. Some of the more important overall areas are contained in the questions that follow: Is your diet more plant than animal based? Do you know about and choose foods based on the Food Pyramid (a good assortment of grains, vegetables, fruits, skim milk, fish, lean meat, poultry, and beans)? Do you choose foods low in saturated fat and sugar? Do you monitor your use of salt? If you drink alcohol, do you do so in moderation?

If you're doing most of these things most of the time, pat yourself on the back! If not, and your goal is to lose weight, you may want to incorporate these suggestions into your eating habits.

Know about Portions, Calories, and Fat

To lose weight, you can a) decrease your intake (calories, fat, portion size); b) increase your output (exercise); or c) do both. The best results come when you do both, plus you receive extra health benefits from exercise that will be discussed in the next section. You will need to monitor what you eat, at least for a while, to determine the amount of calories that you take in currently. There are a variety of weight-loss programs that provide easy systems for monitoring fat and calorie grams. But you can also do it yourself with a few tools. To maximize your learning, you will need: a notebook to write down what you eat, a guide to calories found in a bookstore or supermarket, a food scale that can be purchased inexpensively at a discount retail store, and a set of measuring cups.

Now, for some period of time (at least one "typical" week), use these tools to discover how many calories and fat grams you are consuming. The first week, simply write down what you eat. The second week, pay attention to the serving sizes you consume. The measuring tools (food scale and cups) will help you learn the size of one ounce of meat and the amount of a half-cup of cereal. The third week, write down the calories you eat next to what you ate. You will use the information that you learned about serving sizes to more accurately count the calories you consumed. The fourth week, count the grams of fat that you consume and compare them to your weekly goal.

Tracking what you eat is sometimes difficult, but some people say that this technique is the single best tool for helping them lose weight and stay on track.

How do you figure out how many calories you should consume to begin to lose weight at a rate of one pound per week? There is a scientific formula that compares your calories to your energy expenditure that is a little complex for our purposes here. But there's also a simple, quick way to get a similar result: A pound equals 3500 calories, so if you reduce your calorie consumption by 500 per day, you'll lose a pound a week. Calories burned in exercise contribute to reducing the overall total.

You should also figure out your upper limit of daily fat grams. Generally, no more than 25 percent of your total calories should come from fat, with no more than 10 percent from saturated fats and trans-fatty acids. Your limit should be the number of calories you consume multiplied by .25 divided by 9. Learn more about the types of fat online in the *Dietary Guidelines for Americans* (see Resources).

Although some of this information has probably been review for you, you now know general guidelines for a healthy weight and how to figure out your calorie and fat gram limits to lose weight. Read on for ways to evaluate the reasonableness of your exercise goals.

Create the Right Exercise Plan

You must check with your doctor before beginning any exercise program. Physical activity can help you lose weight, but research shows additional health benefits that can come from regular exercise. There are several different types of exercise. Aerobic activities, which increase heart rate and strengthen the heart muscle, include running, bicycling, swimming, and fast walking. Some exercises increase flexibility, such as stretching and yoga. Some exercises increase muscle strength; these include weight training and isometric exercises. Weight-bearing activities, such as walking, may help strengthen bones.

The types of exercise you can incorporate into your life are endless. Find activities you like to do. Walking is easy and can be done without equipment. You can monitor how much you walk in a typical day by purchasing a pedometer, a small device you can wear at the waist around a belt or clothing. Any activity counts, so look for ways to increase your movement throughout the day, such as climbing stairs instead of taking the elevator or just moving more while doing you usual activity.

Here's the good news. According to the *Dietary Guidelines for Americans* and recent published studies, thirty minutes of moderate physical activity per day is enough to obtain health benefits. Moderate activity is defined as the energy it takes to walk two miles in thirty minutes. This amount may or may not be enough to lose weight. Increasing the intensity of the activity and/or lengthening the amount of exercise time will expend more calories, further strengthen your heart and bones, and lower your risk for cardiovascular disease, colon cancer, and type 2 diabetes. However, new information from the National Academy of Sciences suggests sixty minutes per day is necessary for weight control (see Resources).

Now you can incorporate the guidelines into your health goals to make them reasonable and doable. Revisit the goals you wrote down earlier and revise them if necessary. Check to see that your goals fit your overall life plan, and are reasonable, well-stated, and measurable. Remember, goals that follow these rules can be sustained for the long haul.

Why Are You Getting off Track?

There are many reasons you can stray from your goals. Below are some of the more common reasons you may want to review.

Your Actions Don't Match Your Goals

When your actions don't match your goals, it's likely you'll veer off track. It is usually helpful to return to the big picture to review your overall priorities and the original reasons you had for the goals you created. Return to the Pro-Con Balance Sheet in chapter 1 to help you reflect on your current priorities and readiness to change. Then, think about your overall game plan. Health goals are very important. Be sure that you're doing what's best for you in the long run.

Your Goals Are Not Yours

At times, you may set goals that don't truly come from you, but appear to satisfy other people in your life. The result is usually resentful feelings toward others (or toward yourself if you feel that you "should" accomplish the goals). Not meeting the goals you set is a way of expressing your displeasure at the people you feel are "making" you set the goals, but ultimately sabotages your health. Return to the beginning and think clearly about what you want to do. Revise your goals so that they work for you.

You Feel Restricted by Your Goals

Goals should help you feel positive and motivated. If you feel restricted by your goals, then perhaps they are too stringent or unreasonable. Review the information presented in this chapter about setting good goals. It is also possible that you have a long pattern of indulging yourself when it isn't in your best interest. Read chapter 6 for some strategies to combat this tendency.

You Do Too Much at One Time

You may be excited about your commitment to your health and try to do everything at one time. Resist the temptation to be "good" and hurry through the exercises in this book. If recording your intake for one week is what is suggested, simply do that—don't worry about doing more or being faster. Remember that you will accomplish your plan with reasonable goals and small steps along the way.

Strategies for Staying on Track

The following strategies can help you stay on track with setting and achieving your goals:

1. Set aside a regular time each week to review your goals.

2. Display your written long- and short-term goals in a place where you will see them daily.

3. Schedule your daily tasks according to your long-term priorities.

4. Use visual methods of tracking your progress, such as a graph of your weight loss.

5. Reward yourself for meeting milestones toward your goals.

6. Find creative ways to remind yourself that slow and steady progress will win over the quick and easy route.

7. Read the rest of the book chapters for more ideas for staying on track with your goals and your game plan.

Are Your Hidden Agendas Keeping You from Your Goals?

Many approaches to self-change provide you with a prescriptive, step-by-step plan for what you should be doing to reach your desired goals. There seems to be an assumption that you'll maintain a consistent and reliable focus on what these diet and fitness authorities have told you to do. Unfortunately, when people lose focus, they often ask "why" simply out of frustration, and not with the intent of really understanding the factors that lead them off track. *"Why haven't I gotten on that treadmill I bought?" "Why did I eat that?" "Why did I let the whole evening go without taking a walk?"* Many people simply drop the work out of frustration or return to their game plan no better prepared to deal with the next time they get off track.

In many cases, you have very real reasons and motives for acting counter to your goals. We call these reasons or motives *hidden agendas*. Armed with a new understanding of your hidden agendas, you'll be guided to other chapters of the book to learn how to directly address and manage them.

What Is a Hidden Agenda?

Many of the tasks and duties on your daily agenda are easily identified and apparent to you: pick up the children, finish your report for work, or make dinner. Hidden agendas aren't so apparent. They are more private, personal needs and motives that operate behind the scenes of your busy life. Your hidden agendas can help explain why you snacked late at night, had a second helping, or skipped your workout for a couple of days.

Hidden agendas often come from your very basic needs. Examples include the need to get away from physical discomfort, avoid uncomfortable and anxious feelings, avoid conflict with others, or have consistency and security in your life. Hidden agendas aren't dark or destructive. They can be very real and important concerns to you. However, these agendas cause problems for you when they lead you to do things that are counter to your goals.

Why call it a hidden agenda? Because chances are you don't pay attention to those agendas that steer you off track. Your hidden agendas have likely been around for a long time and acting on them has become like an automatic habit. You may not have learned to be mindful of your personal needs and agendas because you learned to over-focus on the needs of others. Or, you may not be aware of your needs and agendas due to a history of your needs not being acknowledged or openly discussed, or because you did not think you could effectively address them. The word "agenda" is used to emphasize the point that whatever we do, there is typically a reason and purpose. The agendas that we are often most effective at handling are typically those that we are clearly aware of and that we know the reasons for addressing.

A critical assumption here is that your actions, even when counterproductive, are quite understandable when you know the motivations and reasons behind them. Don't worry, this isn't psychoanalysis, and you don't want to start questioning everything you do. The agendas and responses that are of interest here are just the ones that may be interfering with your healthy lifestyle goals. Uncovering your hidden agendas will help you to finally answer the frustrating question, "Why did I do that?"

How Are You Doing Now?

The following types of hidden agendas are commonly seen when people act counter to their exercise and nutrition goals. One or more of the following agendas may apply to your situation. The questions after each example are designed to help you assess whether that particular hidden agenda is disrupting your attempts to change.

The Need to Be Free of Physical Discomfort

No one likes to feel physical discomfort. Unfortunately, losing weight and exercising often involve some form of physical discomfort. During weight-loss efforts, a common discomfort is hunger. Whether it is a slight rumble in the stomach or gnawing hunger pangs, many people are quick to take notice of the hunger and want the feeling to go away immediately. There are weight-loss programs designed to eliminate any feelings of hunger, yet some people still worry about or fear the very *idea* of feeling hunger. Exercise can also produce many types of physical discomfort. Discomfort may come from the pounding on your feet while running, the burning of hard-working muscles, or feeling your lungs reach deep for breath. While many people report a euphoric feeling associated with exercise, many others focus on the uncomfortable feelings involved, and never stick with it long enough to feel the positive sensations.

Now you have two agendas on your plate: the desire to avoid hunger and discomfort, and the desire to have a healthier lifestyle. Unfortunately, you may jump to take care of the physical discomfort without considering the impact to your healthy goals. Do you eat or snack impulsively? This eliminates the hunger, without allowing you any time to consider more thoughtful options. Impulsive eating can also sabotage your exercise goals, as exercising on a full stomach is unpleasant and can cause stomach cramps. Other strategies to avoid the discomfort of exercise may include telling yourself that you will do it tomorrow, simply forgetting about it, or getting distracted by other activities.

What is causing you to quickly resolve your physical discomfort, even though it is working against your healthy goals and what you believe is best for you? A good guess is centered on your thoughts about the discomfort. Are you thinking, "I'm starving," "I'm too tired," "I have to make this go away," or "I can't stand this feeling"? These thoughts may lead you to believe that the discomfort you are feeling is so bad that you should avoid it at all costs, even if it means compromising your goals. The urgency of these thoughts can also make it difficult to consider your health goals and to choose how you want to respond.

The following questions will help you identify whether the need to avoid physical discomfort is an underlying agenda for you. You are encouraged to think about each question and reflect on past incidents where you got off track.

- How quickly do I look to alleviate feelings of hunger and tiredness?

- How well do I tolerate discomfort, while still being able to make careful decisions?

- Do I often give myself permission to immediately satisfy any physical discomfort?

- How often do I tolerate feelings of discomfort in order to continue doing something that I feel is more important?

If you believe that avoiding physical discomfort is an underlying agenda for you that you aren't directly or effectively managing, you are encouraged to pay special attention to chapter 6, Do You Have to Have it Now?. In addition, chapter 5, Where's Your Focus? will help you strengthen your focus and mindfulness skills and help you effectively manage distractions.

The Need to Get Away from Uncomfortable Emotions

In addition to the aversive physical discomfort of tiredness and hunger, there are a number of emotions and feelings that many people are eager to avoid experiencing. Such emotions include anxiety, loneliness, frustration, boredom, and sadness. Whether or not you realize it, how you react to and deal with these feelings can have an unintended impact on your exercise and eating game plan.

These emotions have something in common: they don't feel good and, if possible, most people would choose to feel something different. Problems come up when your escape from the negative feelings happens at the expense of your weight-loss or exercise plans. Impulsive snacking or overeating does address the agenda of temporarily getting rid of negative feelings. The eating gives immediate pleasure and creates a number of new sensations (for example, smell, taste, fullness in stomach) that can distract from or replace the negative feelings. Unfortunately, the negative feelings usually return some time later, often accompanied by guilt and shame. Nonetheless, eating does serve as an immediate relief from the uncomfortable emotions.

We usually have understandable reasons for having the emotions that we do. Unfortunately, we don't always have the skills it takes to deal with negative emotions, and we may try to avoid them at all costs. You may have seen your parents go to great lengths to avoid negative feelings using alcohol, denial, or other avoidant strategies, such as overworking. You may have learned to use food to adjust how you were feeling. These experiences can teach you that negative emotions are intolerable, should be resolved quickly, and need not be addressed directly. Unfortunately, this belief doesn't give you the opportunity to learn how to identify and effectively manage these emotions.

Answer the following questions to help determine whether this is an important hidden agenda for you:

- How frequently do I use food to soothe and comfort myself when I'm feeling bad?

- Do I tend to address uncomfortable feelings, or quickly try to make them go away?

- How would I describe my ability to tolerate negative emotions?

- Does my adherence to my exercise and eating game plan depend on my mood and emotional state?

If this does appear to be a significant hidden agenda for you, you may want to pay special attention to chapter 7, Are Your Unruly Emotions Ruling Your Life?. You will learn more about how you may use food to regulate your emotions, and you'll learn specific ideas for how to directly address and effectively manage the negative emotions. Chapter 6, Do You Have to Have it Now?, will offer advice on how to think through uncomfortable moments to make the best decision for you.

The Need for Autonomy

All adults want to feel like they are in control and in charge of their own lives. The decisions you make about your body and health are yours and yours alone. No one can make you do something that you don't want to do. The reality is that a wide range of external influences can affect your eating and exercise decisions. Opinions from doctors, family, friends, and the media are among the possible sources telling you what you should be doing. Getting feedback from others about what you should do can be a very smart thing. However, if the resulting eating or exercise game plan conflicts with your sense of autonomy and living your life as you see fit, then there could be a problem.

An important factor in successful change is to take ownership of the goal and the necessary work. By owning the goal, you are taking a perspective in which you believe that the goal and results are for you, you take full responsibility for the work, and you are in charge of whether you will continue to pursue the goals. External influences can be effective in creating change in nutrition or exercise habits, but you need to check for feelings of rebellion that can sabotage your change efforts. Is it your goal, your choice, and your responsibility? Do you feel free to stop the work if you choose?

Do you tend to see input from others as intrusive and a threat to your freedom to choose for yourself? If you don't believe the goal is under your control, you may ignore feedback from others or simply drop the goal. Alternatively, you may find yourself so influenced by the opinions of others that you have a rebellious reaction, such as binge eating in secrecy. In either case, there is a perceived threat to your sense of freedom and control, and you respond in an impulsive, counterproductive manner. While it is counterproductive to the eating or exercise game plan, it is quite consistent with your hidden agenda.

Answer the following questions to help you determine whether protecting your autonomy is an important hidden agenda for you:

- Do I think of my exercise or eating game plan as something *I have to do,* as if it is not of my own free choice?

- How often do I feel angry and/or resentful about sticking with my game plan?

- Do I recognize for whom am I doing this?

- Do I find my eating and exercise decisions to be intertwined with issues of power and control with others?

If you think that you're standing up for your sense of freedom and control in ways that are contrary to your healthy goals, this is likely an important hidden agenda for you. Chapter 1, Are You Ready for Change?, will be helpful in recognizing your own reasons and motivations for change. In addition, chapter 2, Are Your Goal and Game Plan Right for You?, discusses the importance of taking ownership of your goals, and chapter 4, Do You Accept the Responsibility for the Choices You Make?, addresses your responsibility to your own goals. Finally, issues of conflict and power with others may accompany your autonomy concerns. Chapter 9, Who's Supporting You?, will help you address conflict and power difficulties.

The Need to Avoid the Risks of Getting Healthier

At first glance, this hidden agenda may seem to make no sense. What kind of risks could you possibly face by exercising and improving your eating habits? Your energy will pick up and your body will thank you. So what's the problem?

There can be risks to getting healthier, depending on how you view the results and the implications of what happens next. For example, there may be uncertainty and fear about moving on to make additional changes in your life. As you feel stronger and more confident, you may want to join a recreational sports league, apply for a better job, or work on expanding your friendships. New goals and challenges can be accompanied by additional anxiety and apprehension. The anxiety may relate to not being sure if your new ventures are the right thing to pursue, exposing yourself to possible failure or being critically judged by others.

Another risk in getting healthier is that your new lifestyle could have a negative impact on important relationships in your life. Building on the success of your healthy goals, your new goals or pursuits may conflict with how others see you and your role in life. For example, a spouse may feel threatened in response to your climb up the corporate ladder, and family members may not like having to redistribute household responsibilities and change schedules and dining habits to adapt to your changing needs. How you think of your ability to successfully address such conflicts will likely determine your perception of risk.

A final example of a risk to getting healthier is that change can upset your desire for familiarity in your life. Many people just like to know that life will be familiar, predictable, and reliable. Becoming healthier, increasing energy, and mobilizing your motivation and drive may represent a loss of consistency and predictability. For some, there is a security and safety that comes from a sedentary lifestyle. Nothing ventured, nothing gained . . . but nothing lost as well.

This hidden agenda centers on protecting yourself from the risks that may occur if you feel healthier and take on new changes and challenges. How do you then respond to these perceived risks? Robert Leahy (1999) discusses "self-handicapping strategies" that people use to inhibit self-improvement efforts and thereby help avoid potential risks and losses. Self-handicapping strategies include staying withdrawn and isolated, procrastinating on exercising, staying distracted with other activities, and overfocusing on physical discomfort. These behaviors can serve to keep you down and protected from the risks that come with living your life in a more full and active style.

Answer the following questions to help you determine whether this is an important hidden agenda for you:

- What makes me apprehensive about taking on new challenges?

- How might my life change if I were to feel stronger and healthier?

- How would I describe my ability to deal with potential changes in my life?

- How important is familiarity and avoiding risks to me?

If this hidden agenda strikes a chord with you, see chapter 1, Are You Ready to Change?, for the advantages and disadvantages of change and self-efficacy beliefs. Strategies for dealing with how your self-improvement will impact your relationships are addressed in chapter 9, Who's Supporting You?. Chapter 8, How Do You Treat Your Mistakes?, will be helpful if you view mistakes, setbacks, or potential criticism as risks to avoid.

The Need to Escape Feeling Deprived

Your day is busy. You give your all at work. You give to your family and friends. Throughout the day, you distribute your time, energy, commitment, and hard work. You may be directing this giving toward everyone but yourself. What may happen is that you get into a pattern of ignoring your needs and wants, which creates a feeling of depletion or deprivation. You may recognize feelings of hunger, tiredness, emptiness, or feeling spent, yet underlying these feelings is a perception of having your needs neglected. People can endure feeling deprived for only so long. At some point, your desire to feel pleasure, comfort, or indulgence in something just for you will become a priority, or hidden agenda. How often do you check in with your personal needs and wants? Do you find yourself having periods of feeling depleted or deprived?

If this is your pattern, when you finally react to feeling deprived, you may give yourself quick permission to indulge in a favorite treat, have a big meal, or postpone scheduled exercise. The thought may be "Hey, I deserve it" or "I gotta give myself a break sometime." No one is saying that you *don't* deserve a break. But this type of giving to yourself is not much of a gift. While you may feel temporary relief, it is often followed by guilt, regret, or anger. What you need is mindful awareness as to how depleted you are feeling, and attention to your emotional and physical needs before you end up in the deprivation zone.

How do you know if you're seeing yourself as depleted? One thing to do is to look at your thoughts about yourself and what you are getting from others when you are tempted to give an impulsive "gift" to yourself.

Some people who had a childhood in which their emotional needs were neglected may have long-standing beliefs that they won't get what they really need in this world. Whether your thoughts are based on recent or chronic feelings of being deprived of what you want, your hidden agenda may be to quickly provide some relief to this feeling. Unfortunately, using food and putting off exercise are short-lived gifts that run counter to your long-term healthy goals.

Answer the following questions to help you identify if avoiding feelings of being deprived is an important hidden agenda for you:

- How well do I balance my personal needs with the needs of others?

- Do I feel that my needs are neglected?

- Do I often feel spent prior to getting off track from my goals?

- Do I impulsively eat as a way to give something to myself?

- How often do I feel like I'm running on empty?

If this hidden agenda seems related to your own experiences with getting off track with your goals, you will be interested in the importance of giving to yourself as discussed in chapter 10, Do You Know How to Make Good Habits a Part of Your Life? As problems with feeling deprived are often related to expectations of yourself, chapter 9, Who's Supporting You?, will be of particular interest. Finally, developing your skills to delay gratification and thoughtfully addressing your needs is strongly recommended, which is the focus of chapter 6, Do You Have to Have It Now?

The Need to Avoid Conflict

For some people, a need to avoid conflict, negative feedback, or anyone being upset with them becomes a high priority. Attending to this agenda can affect close relationships, your ability to stand up for yourself, and work satisfaction. In addition, avoiding conflict can become a hidden agenda that derails your exercise and eating game plan.

For many people, eating and exercise don't take place in isolation from others. Food is prepared by others or eaten with others, meals are planned and food is bought with others in mind, and exercise is scheduled with consideration to family responsibilities. When a high priority is placed on the need to please others and avoid any criticism or negative feedback, you run the risk of being accommodating to others at the expense of your personal goals. For example, you may take seconds so you don't risk offending the cook, postpone exercise to help someone out, or give in when a friend pleads with you to have a dessert with him or her.

Do you find yourself working hard to please and to prevent any problems with others? Conflict is a tricky part of many relationships and it is quite possible that the discussion of conflict in this book could be of some help in other areas of your life. Think hard about how pleasing others, avoiding criticism, and not wanting to upset anyone may interfere with your eating and exercise plans.

Answer the following questions to help you identify whether avoiding conflict is a hidden agenda that may be interfering with your healthy goals:

- Do I tend to forgo exercise to spend time with or help others?

- How much are my eating decisions influenced by the input of others?

- How uncomfortable am I when others don't show approval for healthy habits?

- How quickly do I anticipate criticism or conflict from others?

If your responses indicate that this hidden agenda is relevant for you, chapters 5 and 9, Where's Your Focus? and Who's Supporting You?, are for you. In addition, you may need to brush up on your responsibility to yourself, as discussed in chapter 4, Do You Accept Responsibility for the Choices You Make?

How Can You Be More Successful?

Successfully addressing your hidden agendas will require you to identify and catch them in action. Strategies for effectively dealing with the particular agendas are covered in later chapters.

Identify Your Particular Hidden Agendas

The key to this barrier is to recognize your own particular reasons and motives for when you get off track with your game plan. A critical factor in being able to do so is to approach this issue with a calm, curious, and objective mindset. Anger, disgust, and getting down on yourself will only keep you farther away from understanding the agenda behind your off-track behaviors.

If you find that you're having trouble identifying hidden agendas or underlying reasons as to why you're getting off track with your change efforts, consider the following questions:

1. What are you repeatedly doing that interferes with or is in place of your exercise and eating intentions?

2. What benefit or gain might you get from doing these off-track behaviors?

3. What function or purpose might these behaviors have for you?

4. What feeling or emotion do you escape from by engaging in these behaviors?

5. What are you focusing on that may leave you too depleted to attend to your own health goals?

Catch Your Hidden Agendas in Action

Once you have identified your hidden agendas, you need to "unhide" them. Hidden agendas count on secrecy to survive. If they're identified and well understood, then your logic, reasoning, and problem-solving resources will threaten them. And that is exactly what you want to do. To become more aware of and familiar with your hidden agendas, look for opportunities to see them and remind yourself of their presence. Don't get mad at yourself—simply step back and label the hidden agenda. Calmly acknowledge that while it is quite likely to come up again, you're going to catch it next time. The hiding is over.

In addition to being aware of your hidden agendas, it's also critical to know how you respond to them and end up getting off track with your exercise and eating plans. Typically, your response has satisfied or somehow appeased the agenda. Your responses to the underlying agenda have some valuable effect that reinforces the connection between the agenda and your response. You need to be very aware of your responses that get you off track, and to clearly see the connection between these responses and the underlying agenda.

Be Aware of What Else Is Happening

It will be very helpful to know what else is happening when your hidden agenda is present. How do you know a storm is coming in? The wind picks up, clouds get darker, animals move for cover, and the smell of rain is in the air. These clues tell us that something is brewing and we may want to move for cover. Use the following areas to help you recognize what else is happening at the time that a hidden agenda is being activated.

Thoughts and Images

What are you thinking prior to getting off track? Certain types of thoughts are helpful cues or signs that the agenda is near. "I can't handle it" and "I'm too tired" are great signs that you may be close to doing something that will conflict with your healthy goals.

Emotions and Sensations

What are your feelings prior to getting off track due to a hidden agenda? Many hidden agendas are related to avoiding or getting away from uncomfortable or distressful emotions. You can use the emotions and related sensations to cue yourself to the need to catch the hidden agenda. Strong butterflies in the stomach can direct you to attend to a fear or anxiety, and late-night hunger pangs can be used as a cue to gear up for some important work to keep yourself on track.

Situations and Circumstances

What is happening around you when you act counter to your eating and exercise goals? Are you alone, with certain people, at home? Is there a common time? For many, nighttime is a more difficult time to stay on track. Think about the past circumstances when you got off track and try to identify the factors that seem in common among the situations.

Your thoughts, feelings, surrounding circumstances, and responses can serve as valuable signals directing your attention to hidden agendas. You want to develop a very good understanding of what is happening when your hidden agendas emerge, so you can better recognize and address them.

Why Are You Getting off Track?

The primary source of getting off track with this solution is simply *not recognizing* that your hidden agendas are active and causing you to act counter to your goals. Many people simply don't know about the underlying agenda or motivation steering them off track. Hopefully this chapter has begun to solve that problem for you.

Another explanation for why you aren't attending to your hidden agendas is that you're tying to avoid the uncomfortable feelings that are associated with them. Thinking about hidden agendas, such as uncomfortable feelings, risks of getting healthier, and threats to autonomy, can be very uncomfortable in and of itself. You may feel unsure about what to do or maybe even a bit overwhelmed. You may think of your hidden agenda as another flaw or sign of being defective. A common reaction is to get frustrated when the answers are not coming easily or quickly.

Remember, if it were simple and easy to recognize your hidden agendas, then we wouldn't need to call them hidden. They have developed for a reason, and they aren't going to go away overnight. Your agendas will need to repeatedly be brought out into the light and effectively addressed. As the chapters of this book are designed to help you stay on track with your healthy goals, you can also apply them to staying on track with your hidden agendas.

Strategies for Staying on Track

The following strategies will be helpful in staying on track with recognizing your hidden agendas.

Manage the Negative Emotions

Many of the common hidden agendas have some uncomfortable feeling associated with them. As you recognize the agendas, it will be important to keep any negative emotions at a tolerable or manageable level. Look to chapter 7 for specific strategies to manage unruly emotions.

Address the Hidden Agenda Directly

Many of the chapters of this book are designed to help you directly deal with your hidden agendas. Stay hopeful and remind yourself that you do have resources and can learn how to effectively deal with these underlying agendas.

Don't Lose Your New Understanding

Once you understand your hidden agendas, don't let yourself forget them or pretend they don't exist. You've worked too hard to identify them. The next three suggestions will help you maintain your awareness.

Keep a Log

Record your thoughts, feelings, and the situation in which you may have acted on a hidden agenda. Don't journal about it or write a paragraph. Write down brief descriptions that you believe are directly related to and reflective of the hidden agenda. The more entries you put in, the more familiar and aware you will be of your hidden agendas.

Use Visual Reminders

As discussed, your hidden agendas and their related thoughts and feelings have an automatic, out-of-mind quality. Visual reminders can be very helpful to raise awareness and bring these concerns to the forefront of your mind. Reminder notes, index cards, or any creative means should be put in strategic locations based on the times and situations where the agenda is likely to present itself.

Tell Someone

Choose a friend, family member, or someone you feel will respond in a supportive manner. They don't have to do anything but listen and hopefully offer some encouragement. By telling this person of your hidden agenda, you are bringing it out in the open. You send a strong message to yourself that you don't have to be embarrassed or keep it hidden, but that it is simply a problem to address directly and openly.

Do You Accept Responsibility for the Choices You Make?

Responsibility. Is this more of the parental advice we've all heard since we were children? In a way, yes. The tried-and-true principle of responsibility applies to the many choices you have about eating and exercise in your day. Not recognizing or deflecting responsibility for these choices can become a hidden barrier to reaching your goals. By effectively taking responsibility for your choices, you'll be in the driver's seat as you move toward your goals.

What Is Taking Responsibility for Your Choices?

Achieving your weight-loss and exercise goals will be determined by the actions you take. Whether you are twenty pounds overweight and looking to change your eating habits or two hundred pounds overweight and pursuing surgical treatments, you still have an array of choices related to staying on track with your goals. And for every action you choose to take, there were alternatives you didn't take. The central premise of this chapter requires that you recognize and accept that you almost always have a choice in what you do. Whether you acknowledge it or not, you are responsible for what you choose to do and how you handle the consequences. When you master the skill of taking responsibility, you assume responsibility for your part, no matter what the outcome, and blame no one else. By taking responsibility, you assume maximum control over the success of your weight-loss and exercise goals.

For weight-loss and exercise goals, you are faced with numerous choices about what to do throughout the day. These *moments of choice* typically present an option of adhering to your game plan or choosing an alternative action. Some of your choices about eating and exercise are quite apparent and clear to you. Do you order the steak or the grilled chicken? Do you stop at the gym or go directly home after work? The good news is that you can decide and determine what you will do. The bad news is that if you regret your choice, there is no one to blame but yourself. With every choice, you reaffirm that you own this work—and that the outcome lies squarely on your shoulders.

Other moments of choice are not so apparent but every bit as important. Your actions may come so quickly or automatically that you miss your chance to make a choice about what to do. For example, when you eat late at night, you are repeatedly choosing to take the next bite. However, you probably didn't make a conscious choice to have another bite each time. When did you decide to continue to eat everything that was on your plate? You may be frustrated by a habit of ignoring your morning alarm and missing your scheduled workout time. If so, do you recognize your decision to hit the snooze button on the alarm? Just as ignorance of the law is not a defense, neither is letting yourself think that you aren't choosing each action you take.

Why is taking responsibility for your choices and actions so critical to achieving your goals? First, *someone needs to be in the driver's seat*. There will always be tempting alternatives, unexpected changes, and frequent challenges to sticking with your game plan. Maintaining responsibility for your choices and actions puts you in control of how you will choose to address these moments. Secondly, *your success will require frequent repetitions of the new habits*. Your sense of responsibility becomes stronger through repetition and reinforcement. The more you act responsibly toward your choices, the more likely this behavior will turn into a lasting habit. Thirdly, *you will build strength, confidence, and pride by taking responsibility*. Remember the phrase, strength through adversity? Taking responsibility is often not the easy road. It requires self-awareness and discipline to overcome tempting distractions, excuses, or the tendency to let yourself off the hook. When you take responsibility, you give yourself the message that you are in control and can directly address all the choices presented to you, especially the difficult ones. And lastly, *you won't buy into the myth of not having choices*. If you're taking responsibility for your choices, you won't believe that you had no choice, that things "just happened." This is a dangerous perspective. When you act as if you have no choice or responsibility, your goals are at the mercy of outside influences.

Does This Mean It's All Your Fault?

Absolutely not. Don't confuse taking full responsibility for your choices with being solely to blame for the outcome of your efforts. For example, you typically work a long day, get the children to bed, and find yourself exhausted at 9:30 P.M. It isn't fair or accurate to sum up this example with, "You simply do not choose to exercise at night". The challenges to staying on track, such as other priorities, cravings, tiredness, and stress, are very real and will impact the process. In addition, other factors, such as genetic predisposition, hormones, physical illness, and family, also impact your eating and exercise behavior. However, these influencing factors don't diminish your responsibility to yourself. In fact, taking responsibility for your choices and actions takes place *while* these other influences are affecting you. Challenge yourself to take full responsibility for just your contribution and don't blame yourself for what you can't control. And be mindful of the difference, as a well-known prayer goes.

How Are You Doing Now?

How much responsibility do you take for your choices and actions regarding your healthy goals? This may seem like a loaded question, as we all have a bias toward seeing ourselves as responsible adults. However, the intent here is to just get a clear, accurate picture of yourself.

Read the following statements and check off the ones that describe you:

☐ I often act on "automatic pilot" and don't really feel that I'm in control of my eating and exercise decisions.

☐ I can go days before I stop and question why I have gotten off track with my healthy goals.

☐ I am quick to recognize a lapse in my game plan, but I usually don't think about it until much later.

☐ I tend to attribute my mistakes and lapses to my busy schedule, events, or other situational factors.

☐ If I think my healthy goals will be in jeopardy, I don't usually think ahead and make adjustments to my game plan.

☐ When I am overeating or putting off exercise, I will often find a way to distract myself or justify what I am doing.

☐   I find that I am much more responsible to the needs of others than to my own.

If several of these statements described you, it is likely that you'll benefit from working on this solution. In addition to answering the questions above, you can learn more about yourself by examining your choices and actions when you're getting off track with your game plan. Did you make a conscious decision to not exercise? How did you come to have the second helping? How did you bypass your awareness of the choice you had? Getting off track can teach you a great deal about what is actually happening in your mind when you are making choices that you will later regret.

How Can You Be More Successful?

One approach to taking responsibility for your choices is to simply tell yourself, "Be responsible. I have a choice here. It's up to me!" This quick reminder cuts right to the heart of the matter and may be all you need at times. This section offers you additional suggestions and strategies for how to take responsibility successfully.

Develop a Positive Mind-Set of Responsibility

An important determinant of how well you take responsibility is your thoughts and beliefs about doing so. While everyone can say they believe responsibility is important, you need your own personalized beliefs about responsibility for your choices. A positive mind-set will incorporate: 1) the importance of exerting control over your choices and actions, 2) the value to your self-confidence and self-reliance, and 3) the impact to the success of your goals. Write down a list of your own beliefs about responsibility, incorporating the above themes. The following are examples that you may want to use or adapt for yourself:

- Accepting responsibility for choices has led me to meet goals in the past.

- I want my children to know the importance of taking ownership of their choices.

- Following my game plan almost always feels better to me in the long run.

- I like knowing that I can rely on myself to follow what is really important to me.

- I don't like it when others deflect responsibility, and it isn't okay for me to do it either.

- There is a lot in life I can't control, but I can control what I choose to do.

- As a kid, responsibility felt like something I had to do. Now it's really just part of being good to myself.

- Taking responsibility is taking ownership of what happens in my life; I'm in control of myself.

Use these beliefs and create your own beliefs about responsibility for choices. The beliefs should be positive and ring true for you. You won't be moved by a positive thought that seems superficial or naïve. Look for current evidence that supports the belief. You can also look to past experience, logic, and your rational thinking to confirm the wisdom of your responsibility mind-set.

Recognize All Your Moments of Choice

As discussed earlier, some moments of choice will be very apparent to you and some will not. You need to train yourself to recognize all of them. However, those that are not as easily identified will likely give you more trouble. Times of low energy, tiredness, and tension will likely be high-risk periods where you may have difficulty being mindful of the choices in front of you. The following situations highlight the many moments of choice you may have in your day: feeling stressed at work and recognizing that you haven't had lunch, feeling bored and tired at night and thinking of a snack, or finishing your favorite T.V. show and sitting through the commercials as the next show begins, rather than turning the set off.

These situations illustrate how your days are full of moments when you may or may not take control of what will occur next. You may use a quick justification or go on automatic pilot to do what is easiest or of least resistance. Taking responsibility is a skill whereby you stop and recognize these moments of choice and the potential impact on your game plan.

To help you recognize these moments of responsibility, try using the following steps:

Step 1: Stop and Catch the Moment

Say "STOP" loudly in your head when you recognize that you have a choice and your subsequent actions are going to impact your goals. The "stop" serves to highlight that you have a choice to make. It also interrupts any automatic habit that would allow you to ignore or miss this moment.

Step 2: Acknowledge and Describe What Is Happening

Now that you have recognized the moment, you'll need to understand what is happening and what your responsibility is to yourself. Clearly own up to what you're currently doing and why you're doing it. Next, identify the options or choices you have. Remind yourself of your goals and that you have the ability to choose the most helpful response. Don't let yourself off the hook.

Step 3: Make the Choice and Act on It

Each moment of responsibility will have a different set of choices. Examples include: continue eating or find an alternative way of coping with boredom, put off exercise or plan a specific time to exercise, and snack when feeling tense or use other relaxation strategies. Practice making choices that may not be easy, but will feel good in the long run. This is where you get to build confidence and resiliency.

Once you know what course of action is best for you, *do it and do it quickly*. Delaying or putting off action can give you a chance to fall back into old, familiar habits. You may find it helpful to simply "find yourself doing it." This means acting as if you are on automatic pilot, so that you know you'll follow through and avoid the temptation to change your mind.

Learn from the Choice You Made

So, how did things turn out? Looking back, was your choice a good one? With every situation, you have the opportunity to strengthen your sense of responsibility and develop your self-control and your decision-making skills. In order to do so, you are encouraged to:

Identify Your Responsibility for the Bad Times

Be specific and concrete when you identify what you did wrong. Don't use general or vague statements, such as "I blew it" or "I was lazy." These will likely just create bad feelings. Don't discount or minimize what you did that contributed to negative outcomes, but don't exaggerate those actions either. Rather, be specific and instructive, such as, "Next time I'll know to plan my business lunch at a different restaurant."

Identify Your Responsibility for the Good Times

Some people are in the habit of scrutinizing what they did wrong, but don't take responsibility for when they contributed to important successes with their goals. Be specific and accurate when you identify what you did right. Look at what you did and spend a moment to feel proud and reinforce the wisdom of doing it again in the future.

Make Concrete Plans

It is easy to let past experiences slip into the past, without staying accountable to using what you have learned. Find time in the near future to put your insights into practice. Make specific plans of how you will do so.

Accept Responsibility for Other Problems or Issues

As you reflect on your choices and actions, you may become aware of other problems that are interfering with achieving your goals. Many of these problems, such as unruly emotions and conflicts with others, are addressed in other chapters. The problem is not likely to go away on its own. Take time to consider how best to tackle the problem and what other resources or assistance may be helpful.

Appreciate the Challenge

Most people don't like to think of themselves as "irresponsible." It's quite likely that you are most irresponsible with the actions that affect only you. You may go to great lengths to try to be responsible at home, at work, and with your family, but fall short for yourself. This doesn't make you an "irresponsible person," nor does it mean you are lazy or don't really care. Taking responsibility for all of your actions takes time, energy, and persistence. In addition, as will be discussed in the next section, there are often important issues that are causing you to get off track with taking responsibility. Respect yourself and the challenges that you face as you proceed.

Why Are You Getting off Track?

Along with being aware of your moments of choice, it is important to be aware of why you sometimes don't take responsibility for these moments. With greater awareness, you will be able to catch what you're doing and guide yourself back on track. The following are some common factors that contribute to getting off track.

Not Recognizing the Moments of Responsibility

For some, getting off track is easy to do because they simply aren't in the habit of seeing all of the choices in their day. Identifying such moments is a skill, to be practiced and repeated often. You may have developed the habit of not thinking about your choices and going about your day in an automatic, reactive manner. If that's the case, you may need to acknowledge your habit of missing moments of choice and work hard to catch them from now on.

Feeling Tired and Tense

Low energy and tension often trigger snacking and other off-track actions. As discussed in chapter 7, Are Unruly Emotions Ruling Your Life?, eating can be used in an attempt to alleviate these feelings. Making sound decisions takes time, effort, and energy, and you may not feel up to it during your low-energy times. Don't use feeling tired and tense as an excuse, but as a reminder of a challenging situation that will require extra effort.

Blaming Other People or Circumstances

People can be quite creative in how they deflect responsibility from themselves. You may get upset at the person who offered you the tempting food or encouraged you to have seconds. You might blame your workload, children's activities, or other events that make scheduling exercise difficult. It is important to recognize the impact of other factors, but don't use them as an excuse to avoid your responsibility to your goals.

Believing You Don't Control What Happens to You

Some people don't see themselves as being in control of what happens in their lives. If good things happen, they think it was due to dumb luck or someone else. If bad things happen, they may think it was because of fate or situational factors. If you don't think of yourself as largely determining what is happening in your life, you will have difficulty taking responsibility for your choices and actions. Developing a belief that you can control and determine what happens to you is critical to making lasting change.

Making Responsibility Feel Too Bad

Taking responsibility can be quite difficult, depending on how you think and feel about it. If you think of taking responsibility for your choices as a chore, restriction on your freedom, or part of an all work/no play view of adulthood, then you are likely to avoid it. Or if you react to bad choices with emotions of shame, embarrassment, or anger, you are likely making it too uncomfortable. Taking responsibility can also be a lonely task, as it is up to you and you alone. However, it shouldn't make you feel inferior or isolated from others. If taking responsibility feels too bad, refer to chapter 8, How Do You Treat Your Mistakes?, and chapter 3, Are Your Hidden Agendas Keeping You from Your Goals?

Giving Yourself a "Break"

You may believe that avoiding responsibility is somehow being good to yourself. After all, taking responsibility takes time, energy, and focus, and it can be uncomfortable. In a misguided effort to help yourself, you may conclude that you don't need any more things to do and really need to give yourself a break. No one is watching, so you let the moment slide by. Unfortunately, this quick "gift" to yourself is usually no gift at all. In the long run, it makes you feel less effective and leaves you further from achieving your goals. In addition a misguided break can reinforce a view of yourself as fragile and unable to handle the responsibility.

Taking Too Much Responsibility Elsewhere

You have only so much time, energy, and effort available for being responsible. How are you directing these resources? If you were taught or encouraged to focus primarily on the needs and expectations of others, you may have difficulty attending to those choices that affect only you. Whether you didn't learn to value your responsibility to yourself or you just aren't in the habit of doing so, it will be important to strike a balance between your responsibility to others and to yourself.

Henry's Story

Henry was the oldest of four children who grew up in the middle-class area of town. His mother was a restaurant manager and his father was a car salesman. His parents often worked in the evening and Henry was given considerable responsibility for his younger siblings. While he was proud of how he helped the family, he also had little time for friends or after-school activities.

As an adult, Henry described himself as a good family man. He provided well for his family, loved them very much, and spent almost all of his free time with them. Henry would admit that he wasn't very happy in general and was particularly frustrated about being fifty pounds overweight. He had made sporadic attempts to lose weight and exercise, but he never sustained these efforts.

After reflecting upon his choices and actions throughout the day, Henry first realized that he often acted in an automatic, reflexive style. Not even realizing that he had a choice, Henry would jump to the needs and wants of family members, customers, and coworkers. He never thought about all the choices he was making, such as when and how long to help others, what he would eat, whether to take a walk, how to spend his free time. When he overate, he would think of it as one of his few pleasures for himself.

Henry realized that he did have things he wanted for himself. In addition to losing weight, he also wanted to have more friends and find a hobby. He began challenging his automatic reactions and became more aware of the choices that he did have in his day. Over time, he took responsibility for when he was *choosing* to attend to others and made a mindful choice to stick to his weight-loss plan. As he took greater responsibility for his eating choices, he noted that he felt more in control of his other goals. While he still wants to lose a few more pounds, Henry has less of the weight and more of what he wants in his life.

Strategies for Staying on Track

As you gain awareness of where you're getting off track with taking responsibility for your choices, you'll want to know what keeps you on the right track. Consider the following suggestions and try those that seem most relevant to your situation.

It's Your Show

No two ways about it! It is *your* life, and your health and happiness are *your* responsibility. That fact may seem overwhelming at times, but it can also give you a sense of great control. See yourself as the one in charge. Monitor your choices and actions with calm objectivity. Whether the outcome is good or bad, know that you can step up and take responsibility. Use notes and other visual reminders to help you stay mindful of this.

Practice When It's Hard

All skills need to be practiced and strengthened, especially when it is more challenging to do so. Be mindful of your choices when you're tired, at the end of a long workday, or when you're feeling stressed. Or catch yourself right in the middle of deflecting responsibility for a choice. The biggest gains often come from the most challenging work.

Be a Great Coach

The first two suggestions require discipline and making yourself do things you may not really feel like doing. Guiding yourself to do what you may not feel like doing is part of being an effective coach. But so is being very encouraging and supportive. Make sure you are giving yourself instruction that is firm and disciplined, yet supportive. Mix in a good dose of humor and lightness, to make sure you'll want to stick around with this coach.

Do Yourself a Favor

As discussed in the earlier section on the positive mind-set of responsibility, it's important to be mindful of what banishing this hidden barrier can bring to you. You may find it easy to see holding yourself responsible as aversive and restricting. In fact, taking great responsibility for your choices and actions is the surest way to accomplish your goals. In addition, remember the positive impact it can have on your self-esteem and confidence. Maintaining a responsible stance toward your new health behaviors is a favor and a gift to yourself. Practice thinking in this new way.

Practice Responsibility in Other Areas

The responsibility discussed in this chapter isn't restricted to just your healthy goals. In fact, the skills involved in taking responsibility will also impact the success you have in other areas of your life. Use this solution at work, in your relationships, and with your other personal goals. The more you take effective responsibility for your choices, the stronger this behavior will become in all areas of your life.

Address Other Related Problems

The section on getting off track referred to several problems that can interfere with this solution. These issues include being overly responsible for others, blaming others, shame, and low energy. Eating can also be associated with a need for control over something in your life. Are you feeling a lack of control in your relationships or at work? You need to be mindful of how such issues are affecting your progress and stay responsible to see that they get effectively addressed. If outside help is needed, go for it. Such issues don't magically go away, and they may repeatedly interfere with achieving your goals.

Where's Your Focus?

If you're like most people, you face many challenges, including unscheduled interruptions, urgent deadlines, everyday responsibilities, and the occasional upheavals that come with an uncertain world. Focusing on your lifestyle goals and game plan in the midst of these demands isn't always easy. One of the more important skills you need in order to achieve your weight-loss and exercise goals is a keen focus. Not knowing why maintaining focus is hard for you can be a hidden barrier. But how can you focus with so much going on in your life? In this chapter, you'll learn how to develop your ability to consistently direct your attention toward those activities that will assist you the most. You will learn to do so when you feel distracted or aimless, when you've lost direction, or when you just don't feel like following through with your plans.

What Is Focusing?

Focusing on your goals and game plan means that you're able to concentrate your attention and efforts on what is most important to you. It may be helpful to think of focus in two different components: the focus of your attention and the focus of your motivation.

Attentional focus refers to how well you focus on one task at a time and how well you focus on your game-plan strategies. Attentional focus on tasks is the type of in-the-moment concentration you need when you are completing a project that requires your attention, such as ordering from a menu, choosing a healthy snack, or following your exercise plan for that day. When your attention is good, you concentrate fully on the task until it is completed. When your attentional focus wanes, you are likely to distract yourself with unrelated thoughts or stop what you are doing entirely and move on to something else. Attentional focus on your game-plan strategies refers to how well you concentrate on planning and enacting your game plan in the context of your life. When you have a healthy attentional focus on your strategies, you are aware of your priorities and you choose your actions accordingly. You feel in control of your daily habits when you possess a sense of focus on the long term.

Motivational focus refers to your underlying drive or desire to accomplish your goals. A lack of motivational focus might be expressed as the thought that you "just don't feel like exercising." Your motivational focus will normally wax and wane in intensity at times, but it must be maintained at a minimum level in order for you to follow through with actions.

If you lack one or more of these components of focus, there's good news for you. Each one of the components is a skill that can be developed and strengthened. The importance of focusing on your goal and game-plan strategies cannot be overstated. Losing focus means veering away from the opportunity to achieve your goals. Learning to focus, even during times when it's hard for you, is vital to keeping on track. With the knowledge and practice of the strategies in this chapter, you'll be well on your way to increasing your focus on the lifestyle goals that are important to you.

How Are You Doing Now?

If you aren't sure whether a lack of focus poses a problem for you, read the following statements and check off the ones that describe you best.

☐ I can generally concentrate on one thing at a time.

☐ My desire to pursue my goals is strong and steady.

☐ Achieving my lifestyle goals is one of my highest priorities.

☐ I consistently remind myself of my priorities.

☐ I use strategies that keep my actions focused on my goals.

☐ I am easily distracted by other things I have to do.

☐ My thoughts wander when I try to think about one thing.

☐ My motivation to eat well and exercise comes and goes.

☐ Sometimes I forget my goals and game-plan strategies.

☐ I have trouble maintaining the actions of a healthy lifestyle.

If the first five statements seem to describe you, then a lack of focus may not be one of the primary reasons you veer off track from your goals. You probably maintain the type of focus that will help you attain your healthy lifestyle goals. If the last five statements describe you, then improving your focus may help you stay on track toward your goals.

What Is Getting Your Focus?

Rest assured that you are focusing on something. The question is whether you are aware of what captures your attention in your everyday life. Take a minute to review the activities you accomplished in the last twenty-four hours or look at a typical day's schedule to see what is capturing your focus. You can probably list the activities readily, such as working, sleeping, preparing meals, or caring for children. Were you truly focused on these tasks or did your attention wander to other things, perhaps the next item on your to-do list? How much focus did you put on meeting your healthy lifestyle goals or enacting your daily lifestyle game plan in relation to other activities?

Knowing whether focusing is problematic for you and understanding what is currently demanding your attention will help you identify small moments to address and systematic problems that hinder your ability to focus. You're now prepared to learn more about ways to gain and maintain focus.

How Can You Be More Successful?

To be successful with this solution, you'll need to know some strategies that increase each type of focus. The exercises below will help you develop your ability to concentrate on your goals.

Recognize When You Lack Focus

The more you know about situations in which you're most vulnerable, the better. Think about the last time you were aware of losing focus on your goals and game plan. What were you doing? What was your attention focused on at the time and what distracting factors affected you? Some people have cardinal signs that warn them that they're losing focus. Think about the physical sensations you have when you realize that you aren't focused. Are you restless? Do you feel a knot in your stomach? Think about the overall sense of motivation you have when you lose focus. Do you experience a lack of desire to implement your goals? What actions do you typically take when you recognize that you aren't focused? Your awareness of yourself is very important here. Every person is unique and will therefore have different times and ways in which they are most vulnerable to losing focus. If you don't know the answers to some of these questions, resolve to observe yourself over the next few days and find out more about your tendencies. The more expert you become at knowing when and how you lose focus, the better able you will be to address them with the strategies suggested below.

Learn the Skill of Mindful Focus

Mindful focus is the skill of being aware of what is happening at the moment. The phrase "mindful focus" comes from mindfulness meditation, which is the practice of meditation and awareness of "what is," practiced and popularized by Jon Kabat-Zinn, Ph.D. (1990). The constant stream of thoughts and images in your mind can keep you from a clearer awareness of your personal reality or what is happening in your life at the moment. Try closing your eyes and clearing your mind for five minutes. How long after you closed your eyes did your thoughts begin? When you try to calm your mind deliberately, your mind often moves like a monkey jumping from tree to tree. Thoughts of what you must do right now often appear, as well as thoughts that aren't relevant. Just after you close your eyes, you might begin to think about something you rarely think about, such as whether you turned off the coffee maker that morning. When reassuring yourself doesn't seem to help, you begin to wonder if your kitchen is on fire and suddenly you hear yourself saying, "I can't be here relaxing. My house is on fire!" Another common trick your mind will play as you try to relax is to incessantly remind you of all you have to do. Whether these items are urgent or not, your mind will attempt to convince you that you don't have time to meditate or focus. The sense of urgency behind the jumping thoughts keeps you from focusing on more important issues that aren't going well in your life. These extraneous thoughts may keep you from thinking about an unhappy marriage, broken relationships, or feelings of failure.

Mindful focus involves tuning in to what is happening at this instant. It means being aware of your physical and emotional sensations and the sights and sounds in the environment right now. As you focus, you may tune in to deeper emotions, such as sadness or fear or feelings of unworthiness. You may also be aware of joy or contentment. When you are able to acknowledge what you are experiencing in the moment and "be with" whatever comes in an open and nonjudgmental fashion, you will experience life more fully. A side benefit of mindful focus is that as you concentrate on the moment, your need to be distracted by extraneous thoughts and actions will dissipate. You will have more time and energy to give your full attention to what you are doing in the present.

Developing mindful focus involves practice, generally the practice of deep breathing and meditation. You can increase your awareness right now by stopping what you are doing, closing your eyes, and taking a slow, deep breath. Allow your exhalations to be twice as long as your inhalations. Take a minute to simply allow whatever you notice to enter your awareness. Try not to react to whatever you discover. Just be open and nonjudgmental. If your thoughts pull you away from your meditation, gently acknowledge the thoughts as they come and return your attention to your breathing.

Although the point of mindfulness meditation is *not* to achieve a goal, the skill of mindful focus can be used to help you attend to what is happening at any given moment. Through this practice, you'll heighten your awareness of your current experience and you may gain an awareness of thoughts that are distracting your attention, motivation, or actions. You will find yourself more able to handle the real distraction and to move toward the picture you have envisioned of your success.

Effectively Manage Responsibilities

The busy lives we lead today result in many responsibilities to juggle. That makes it crucial for you to attend to the everyday practicalities of life in a manner that works for you. To effectively manage your responsibilities, you must:

- understand and practice time management

- plan around your priorities

- develop the ability to say "no" (and use it)

- balance your needs with the needs of others

- learn to delegate responsibilities

Time-management skills are crucial to your ability to focus. When you have "too much to do," you may have difficulty identifying which activities are worthy of your time. Most people feel that they don't have enough time. Hyrum W. Smith (1994), time and life-planning expert, puts it this way: Every individual is given a daily check for twenty-four hours. Each of the 86,400 seconds given to you each day must be spent. Therefore, every person has time. Additionally, every person has the same amount of time as everyone else. The lack of time isn't the problem. How you spend your time is what makes the difference. Review your time-management skills according to your values and priorities, and let your overall values and priorities determine your focus for your long- and short-term goals. Daily activities should be undertaken according to these values and goals.

Although planning and prioritizing are crucial, you also need to set up your environment to assist you in meeting your priorities. Arrange things so you have to think as little as possible about routine aspects. One example is to make a list of healthy foods that you want to have in the house on a regular basis. Place these on a standard shopping list and add additional items as they are needed.

Focusing on your priorities and reviewing them on a regular basis should help you distinguish between times you need to say "yes" and times when you should say "no, thank you." If the request, whether it is a volunteer activity or an offer of a tempting food, is not in line with your goals and game-plan strategies, say "no, thank you." Remember that you have to spend your life-seconds wisely.

Children and family responsibilities are often cited as reasons for difficulties with meeting healthy lifestyle goals. Employ creative thinking, and by all means, involve the family to help you think of ways to balance your needs with their needs. If you think that you "have to bring unhealthy food into the house" because your children won't eat anything else, ask yourself what you are teaching them about maintaining their health. Create a family project to find tasty, healthy snacks. If life after school is "too hectic to exercise," involve your children and have a family exercise time.

Learning to delegate responsibilities can also help you focus. Enlist your children to help in whatever ways they can. Even young children can help by picking up their toys. You'll be teaching them responsibility at the same time you're carving out time to meet your healthy lifestyle goals. Organizing the practicalities of your life will help you manage your responsibilities in a way that increases your focus.

Create a Picture of Success

A powerful way to increase your focus is to create a picture of success that you can use at any time to reinforce your goals and game plan. First, create a detailed picture of what it will be like to reach the weight-loss and exercise goals you have created for yourself. Include all of your senses in the picture (how you think and feel, what you see in your surroundings, what you hear people telling you, etc.). Write a paragraph or draw a picture of what it would be like to reach your weight-loss and exercise goals. Second, create a picture of success in achieving your game-plan strategies. Picture yourself exhibiting perfect motivation toward your goal. See yourself exercising when you aren't in the mood and choosing healthy foods in your most vulnerable situations. Keep these paragraphs or pictures somewhere where you will see them on a daily basis. Review them in your mind until they become real. The more you rehearse your success, the easier it will be to focus.

Use a Step-by-Step Process

When you find yourself losing focus on your goals or game plan, use the following step-by-step process to increase your focus:

Step 1: Tune In

Use mindful focus to tune in to what you're feeling when you notice that you're distracted from your goal. Observe what you experience. Isolating what is happening for you at that moment will guide your decisions.

Step 2: Weigh the Priorities and Urgency

The second step involves weighing what to do next in light of your priorities and the urgency of action. Step 1 will likely reveal distracting elements. You may decide to acknowledge what is going on for you and return to focusing on your game-plan strategies. There may be times in which you'll need to delay or stop your plans for healthy eating or exercising because something higher on your priority list takes precedence. You may find a need to do one of three things: a) reprioritize your current activities, b) gently remind yourself to return to focusing on the task at hand, or c) choose to perform some of the solutions in this chapter that enhance your sense of focus. Sometimes mindful focus will reveal hidden agendas or emotions that would likely be resolved if you spent a little time taking care of them. Simply acknowledging your feelings, say of sadness or fear, may be enough for the feeling to dissipate and allow you to focus on your game-plan strategies. Alternatively, you may find you need to spend more time thinking about emotions, hidden agendas, and other ways of veering off track presented in other chapters in this book. To decide whether to stop focusing on your game-plan strategies or continue on, weigh your actions against your priorities and the urgency of each.

For example, pretend that a friend has called you with some unsettling news about her health. You feel upset and disrupted. You are barely able to put your worry aside and finish your work. Although you had planned to stop by the gym after work, you notice that you no longer feel like following your usual routine. You feel like going to bed. Instead, you tune in and notice feelings of anxiety and restlessness. You allow yourself to feel the full impact of your friend's bad news. Now you can decide whether to stick to your plan or change it. As you think through the options, you decide that exercising will help you release the anxiety so you will be better able to support your friend. Having used the skill of mindful focus, you were better able to weigh your priorities. If you had distracted yourself from your present experience, you might have done something that neither met your goal nor helped your friend.

Step 3: Match the Strategy to the Type of Focus

Different types of focus sometimes require different strategies. To increase your attentional focus, practice the skill of mindful focus. Remember to adopt a present-oriented, open attitude toward your awareness in the moment. If you find pressing emotions or agenda items weighing on you, address them only if they are priorities and then return to your focus on your goal and game plan. Try not to reprimand yourself for losing focus, but gently encourage yourself to return to your priority.

To improve your motivational focus, rehearse your success scenarios until they become second nature. When you catch yourself lacking focus, interrupt your lack of motivation by envisioning your success scenarios. Review the Pro-Con Balance Sheet in chapter 1 if you feel a serious lack of motivation. Additionally, review your goals and game plan at regular intervals to be sure they meet your real needs. Write and post a list of positive reasons you are pursuing good health. Ask for words of encouragement from friends and family members if that is helpful for you.

Improving your focus on your actions means paying attention to what you do. Remember that every action counts. When an action seems too complicated, break it into small parts and begin with one small part. Action begets action, so doing anything in the direction of your goals will likely help you feel ready for more action. Try to do one thing at a time with full consciousness. Anticipate and plan for times when following through with your game plan strategies will be difficult. Enlist family members to help you, and delegate when possible. Finally, remember to reward yourself for acting in your best interest.

David's Story

David was an executive with a marketing firm. He worked long hours. He and his wife, Patty, a CPA, decided that she would work part-time from their home while their two children were of preschool age. Since beginning his career ten years earlier, David had gained fifty pounds, which he attributed to his need to entertain customers at fine dining establishments. When his yearly health checkup revealed high blood pressure, he made a goal to lose weight and to increase his daily exercise. However, there were a few difficulties.

First, he found that his plan for going to the gym directly after work wasn't working. He always had more work than he could finish, so leaving work earlier than he had to was frustrating. And Patty expected him home by 8:00 P.M. on nights he didn't have to entertain customers so that he could help prepare the children for bed. Going to the gym after having dinner and putting the children to bed didn't work because by then he felt too tired to exercise. To top it off, he had no idea how he could alter his meals when he took clients out for lunch or dinner.

David identified trouble with motivational and attentional focus. Although he felt overwhelmed, he decided to spend the first fifteen minutes of every morning increasing his motivational focus. This small commitment to action paid off after a couple of weeks of fifteen-minute increments in which he reviewed the pros and cons of changing his exercise and eating habits and realized that reducing his blood pressure and preventing heart disease was very important to him. At the end of a few weeks, he made reasonable goals and an initial game plan. Instead of going to the gym, he increased his activities with small actions, such as parking the car some distance from the office. This added up to about forty-five minutes of walking each day.

To increase his attentional focus, he decided to spend his morning fifteen minutes practicing mindful focus. As he continued his disciplined practice, he learned to use mindful focus to tune in to his circumstances and to relax his muscles when he felt tense. This technique helped him increase his awareness of food choices. Soon he felt confident selecting low-fat lunch and dinner entrees. His new habits took some practice to maintain, but he found that increasing his daily focus on his goals was the key to his overall success.

Why Are You Getting off Track?

When you have trouble implementing the focusing strategies in this chapter, step back and evaluate whether one of these common situations is hindering your efforts.

Overwhelming Responsibilities

One reason you may have trouble focusing is that you feel overwhelmed by your responsibilities. If this is the reason you feel you lose focus, then a thorough overhaul of your priorities and time management skills may be in order. If you feel you can't spend time to stop and reevaluate the big picture, then ask yourself what is keeping you overloaded. Perhaps you have difficulty saying "no." Perhaps feeling overwhelmed is serving some other purpose in your life, such as to distract you from more important matters. You may get something from feeling overly responsible for events and activities in your life. Are you rewarded for having too many responsibilities? You may feel valuable to people when you are very responsible. You may use being overwhelmed to prove to yourself that you're the responsible one in your family. Feeling overwhelmed may also keep you from focusing on more painful tasks, such as addressing a failing marriage. Ask yourself what you gain from allowing yourself to be overwhelmed.

Lack of Energy

Losing focus can come from a lack of energy or rest. As paradoxical as it may seem, moving more can renew your energy. Take a walk, get some exercise, or change your surroundings for a short time when malaise sets in. A short period of relaxation may also help you feel revived and more able to concentrate. When the feeling of low energy is due to your emotions, such as feeling down or blue, try using mindful focus or the techniques in chapter 7.

Food Cravings

At times, a craving for a favorite food may overshadow your attempts to focus on choosing healthy foods. When the favorite food is a healthy one, then indulge yourself! Most likely, however, you will crave high-fat, high-calorie foods. If you crave these foods, first try using mindful focus to ascertain whether you are trying to satisfy another desire with the food craving. Food cravings can be another way your mind keeps you distracted. If your desire for the food doesn't pass and you begin to feel deprived, eat a small amount of the food or try a healthy substitute. For example, cravings for chocolate can often be satisfied with low-fat alternatives, such as low-fat, low-calorie desserts or hot chocolate.

You "Can't" Relax

Sometimes there is so much going on that it feels impossible to relax, which is an important element in improving your focus. There are people who believe that they are physically unable to relax. A common underlying belief is that if you relax, you won't accomplish anything. Actually, anxiety takes up precious energy that you could be using toward attaining the goals you set for yourself.

When you feel too anxious to relax, try breathing deeply. After all, no matter where you are or what you're doing, you have to breathe. So you might as well breathe deeply from your diaphragm. Still not convinced? Think about this: It's physiologically impossible to breathe properly, that is, deeply and from your diaphragm, and be in a state of high anxiety. Next, try focusing on one thing at a time. You may find it necessary to focus on small increments. Soon you'll notice that as you let go of your anxiety, you'll have what you need to concentrate and focus.

Strategies for Staying on Track

To stay on track with your focus on your goals and game plan, try the following strategies.

Brainstorm with Family and Friends

Ask your family and friends to help you be creative in solving some of the practical obstacles you have to maintaining focus. Hold a brainstorming session and ask them to come up with as many ideas as they can. Then, evaluate which ones will work for you.

Try the Techniques, Even When You Don't Feel Like It

The techniques in this chapter will help you the most if you try them when you least feel like it. Don't think about it—just dive in. You'll be surprised at how your focus will return.

Keep Practicing Mindful Focus

Keeping your awareness in the moment is difficult and requires practice. Your practice will pay off in many ways as you learn to pay attention to your experience in the present moment.

Be Willing to Experience Your Thoughts and Feelings

To be mindful in the moment sometimes means experiencing the full impact of your emotions. When the emotions are negative or cause anxiety, it can be difficult to focus on them fully. However, when you learn to do this, you will be better able to focus on implementing your goals and game plan.

Do You Have to Have It Now?

Americans are notoriously impatient. We don't want to wait for anything. Our country is home to fast food and drive-through banking. So, when it comes to our private lives and eating habits, it's no wonder that our general inclination is to indulge ourselves. Why wait if you don't have to? Gratification, preferably immediate, becomes the order of the day. The problem, of course, is that a pattern of instant gratification has its downside. The downside is that instant gratification may not be in your best interest. An inability to stop acting like you must have it, and have it now, is one reason you might veer from your goals. A repeated pattern of instant gratification can be a hidden barrier to reaching your goals. The central strategy offered in this chapter is to help you change your "I must have it now" mind-set and learn to practice patience. A hard fact of life is that you can't meet your goals and simultaneously indulge every craving and desire when you want it. If this paragraph makes you move a little in your seat, feel uncomfortable, or whisper to yourself, "Hey, are they talking about me?," then please continue reading. This chapter on patience is for you.

What Is Practicing Patience?

Practicing patience is the means by which you will learn to pinpoint those moments when you think you *must have* what you want and transform them into opportunities to act in your long-term interest. Practicing patience boils down to small acts that add up to big results over time. It means deciding to act in your own interest no matter what it takes. Does it mean never being able to satisfy your cravings? Absolutely not! It means satisfying your cravings in ways that won't be hurtful to you.

Practicing patience is important because it will help you act on your true needs. The great part is that when you learn to practice patience, you'll become less interested in participating in actions that don't lead toward your goals. For example, you will pass up a dessert with the feeling that you really don't want it or you'll find being sedentary is increasingly unsatisfying. Can you imagine that? It's true. When you understand that there are no quick fixes and you begin to practice patience, you exert control over your life, and that will ultimately bring you satisfaction and success.

How Are You Doing Now?

If you don't know immediately whether instant gratification is a reason you veer from your goals, read the statements below and check off the ones that describe you best.

☐ When I want something, I generally allow myself to have it.

☐ I won't wait long for something I want.

☐ If I want something done, I want it done now.

☐ I indulge myself in unhealthy habits without thinking.

☐ Waiting is torture.

☐ I interrupt myself when I notice I'm about to go against my game plan.

☐ I can wait to get what I want.

☐ I have met a larger goal by taking small steps.

☐ A slow and steady pace fits my lifestyle.

☐ I generally weigh my actions against my overall interests.

If the last five statements seem to describe you best, then the need to immediately satisfy your desires may not be one of the primary reasons you veer off track from your goals. However, if the first five statements describe you better than the last five, then learning to practice patience may help you attain your goals.

How Can You Be More Successful?

The following strategies can help you increase your patience with the process of losing weight and exercising.

Change Your Thoughts

At the heart of patience is the thought, "I don't have to have it right now." With this belief, you are able to calm your urges, engage in other actions, and stay on track with your long-term goals. To build patience, you must catch thoughts such as, "I can't wait" or "I must have it now." Challenging or stopping these thoughts is integral to practicing patience. Different ways to alter your thinking are described in the following sections.

Banish the Rules

If you impulsively engage in poor eating habits and a sedentary lifestyle, you may be like the people who were told to think about anything but a pink elephant. What did they think about? Right. The biggest, pinkest elephant you can imagine. Similarly, when you tell yourself that you "can't eat that" or you "must exercise," guess what happens? Part of you rebels and sneakily answers back, "Oh yeah?" Now, not only *can* you have that thing to eat, you *must* have it. And you tell yourself that you absolutely, positively, *will not* exercise today. You deserve a break, after all!

What's happening here is that you perceive that there are rules that you must follow. Even though you are the one who set the "rules" for your own best interest, you begin to behave as though they were set by an outside source. It's as if you are a teenager catapulted to the past and a parent is telling you what to do. All of a sudden, you perceive the goals and game-plan strategies you created as ones that have been imposed upon you against your will.

The best way to calm the rebel voice is to banish the rules. Rules don't work anyway. There is plenty of evidence to show that barring yourself from the "bad foods" is not helpful. There are no "bad foods." You can have anything. You are in total control of the foods you eat and the calories you expend. Of course, you also have to accept the consequences your choices bring. Can you have anything at any time you want in any amount you want? Absolutely yes . . . if you want to take the consequences. You *can* satisfy your cravings and meet your lifestyle goals if you are creative and committed. If you're craving a donut, eat a donut. Just don't eat two or three. The calories and fat grams count, so write them down and adjust the rest of your intake or increase your energy expenditure. Alternatively, find something healthier to substitute, such as a slice of whole-wheat raisin bread. If banishing all the "rules" you have for achieving a healthy lifestyle is too scary, try experimenting by testing out the ideas presented in this chapter. Many people find that their need to "have it right now" decreases dramatically when they throw away their list of "must-not-have" foods.

Use Your Successes

Somewhere in your life you have achieved something important by taking small steps. Perhaps you lost weight in the past or established an exercise program. Perhaps you completed a project or educational program in a series of small steps. Use your successes to ask yourself what helped you sustain your motivation even when tempted by the prospect of instant gratification. What helped you complete the project instead of watching television? How were you able to avoid instant gratification in the past? What techniques helped you focus on the larger goal in situations where you were tempted to act against your own interests? Perhaps you enlisted the help of others by calling them when you felt tempted. Perhaps you used visualization techniques, such as seeing yourself reaching the goal or imagining how you would feel if you skipped your workout or ate the three donuts on the table. Make a list of what helped you in the past. Brainstorm ways you can use these ideas in your current situations when you may want to react before you think.

Adjust the Pace

A commitment to success sometimes conjures up images of a fast-paced environment, moving at lightning speed, with increased pressure to produce more and more progress toward your goals. Fast-paced environments increase the likelihood that instant gratification is the order of the day. However, success in habit change means being patient with the process, step by step. The father of author Lynette recounts two methods of picking beans on the family farm in the southwest. His father would offer to compete against his children for the fastest time to pick rows of beans. Each child would be poised at the beginning of the row and would exert a lot of energy, hurrying as fast as possible to get the lead in the beginning of the race, only to become fatigued and breathless halfway down the row.

His father, on the other hand, would start off slowly, deliberately picking at a steady pace. He would always beat his children in the picking game. He said he was in a "slow hurry."

What were the differences between the father and his children? The children had expectations of winning. They pumped up the adrenaline in order to win. Their thoughts were more dramatic. They *had* to hurry to beat their father. Their bodies responded to the messages they were giving themselves. Their father, on the other hand, didn't react in this way. There was no drama or urgency in his reaction. He moved at a slow and steady pace while his expectations were that he would prevail. Does one of these styles describe you when you feel like you need instant satisfaction? What are your thoughts when you choose to be patient and move steadily toward your goal?

Adjusting the outward pace of your life may not be easy, although it would likely be helpful. Even if you are unable to make major adjustments to the outward pace of your life, you can adjust your inner pace to a "slow hurry." A steady, deliberate pace with a sense of calm urgency will help you avoid impulsive actions. You can begin to adjust your inner pace by developing a mindful focus, as discussed in chapter 5. When you slow down your mind's constant chatter, you will be less likely to respond to urges for instant gratification.

Make Peace with the Past

Sometimes the tendency toward instant gratification comes from past learning experiences. If you were rewarded by food or learned to manage your emotions by eating, your tendency toward impulsive eating may be greater than if you hadn't had these experiences. You may have witnessed someone in your family who ate to excess, lived a sedentary lifestyle, or participated in unhealthy lifestyle behaviors. Further, these individuals may have rationalized their participation in these activities by saying that they deserved to have what they want. They managed to minimize the consequences of their behavior.

Making peace with a past that reinforced instant gratification isn't easy. Brain chemistry also contributes to the problem by providing a sense of satisfaction after the consumption of high-fat, high-sugar foods. Making peace with the past requires a shift in your thinking and a continued commitment to your goals. Identify the times when you are most prone to acting like you must have it now, and ask yourself whether you are driven by past experience. Are there old messages about instant gratification you are giving yourself that are no longer relevant or that sabotage your long-term health? Tell yourself that you no longer need to listen to these messages. Write a letter (that you don't send) to the people who reinforced the idea that you had to have what you wanted even if it wasn't good for you. Tell them that while you appreciated their motivations on your behalf, you no longer need these messages or teachings. From now on, you will decide on your future. Forgive whomever you need to forgive and let the old messages go. By doing so, you will put yourself in charge of your commitment to your lifestyle goals.

Indulge Yourself

Yes, you read that right. Indulge yourself. Indulge yourself with foods that nourish your body. Reward yourself by creating an active lifestyle. Pamper yourself with positive thoughts about your ability to reach your goals. If you change your definition of indulgence from that which is forbidden to something that's healthy for you, instant gratification doesn't sabotage your goals. Start with healthy foods and exercises you really like. As you begin to concentrate on the pleasure you gain from enacting your game plan, you will become more patient and committed to the daily strategies that will lead you to your goals. Eventually, you may wonder why you were so tempted by high-calorie foods and a sedentary life. Invite yourself to change your definition of what indulgence means, and use the concept to remind you to be good to yourself.

Why Are You Getting off Track?

Common reasons for falling off track when you are learning to practice patience go to the heart of why immediate gratification may be a stumbling block for you. If you find yourself having difficulty interrupting the cycle of instant gratification and practicing patience, see if you can relate to some of the reasons below.

Chronic Feelings of Deprivation

Feelings of deprivation can stem from a variety of sources. You may not feel that you have what you need emotionally or physically. You may feel like you are "not enough," a feeling that you probably got from your past. When you feel deprived, you may react by trying to get what you can and to do it quickly, thus leading to impulsive actions that are the opposite of your game-plan strategies. Acting in an impulsive way becomes a coping strategy that is outdated and unhelpful, even though it may have served a purpose in the past.

Inattention

The drive to satisfy cravings sometimes comes from inattention to your physical needs. Inattention can be a factor when you are overly hungry as well as when you aren't hungry at all. When you don't eat at regular intervals, your physiological feelings of hunger will begin to warn you that it's time to eat. Continued inattention to these sensations may cause you to eat whatever you can, regardless of whether you're following your game-plan strategies. Additionally, you are likely to eat more than you would have if you hadn't been so hungry. Not paying attention to your physical needs can also lead to eating out of habit, without thinking about what you're doing. You may find yourself giving into a craving when you're on automatic pilot, simply because you're not paying attention. Catching yourself when you're not paying attention and changing how you react is important. When you fall off track from your goals repeatedly because of inattention, consider tracking everything you eat for the next week. Plan to implement some of the strategies in this chapter to help you become aware of times you could practice patience.

Fears of Adjusting the Pace

When the habit of immediate gratification is strong, there is often a rushed attitude or "hurry up" demeanor. You may be so used to the fast pace of your activities that you fear that slowing down will interfere with accomplishing your goals. You operate as if urgency is necessary to accomplish anything. Some stress is necessary to accomplish things in life, but it's not true that if you slow down, you will ultimately fail to achieve the goal. If this is a fear of yours, begin in small ways to slow down. You will likely find the opposite of what you fear. That is, when you slow the pace, you have more energy to devote to the task. Anxiety takes energy that you can devote to more productive tasks, like focusing more clearly on your lifestyle goals.

Love of the Party

Another reason you may have trouble with practicing patience is that you may be a person who loves a celebration a little too much. Any day, any event, is declared a celebration and, of course, along with that comes permission to overindulge. Meeting your needs is the order of the moment. When this attitude is taken to an extreme, interrupting the cycle is difficult because it can seem like there will be no fun in life without continuous permission to go all out. If you can relate to this reason for falling off track with your goals, you must decide if what you are gaining is worth the long-term consequences. You don't have to stop celebrating. There are a lot of ways to celebrate using healthy foods. Active events can help you celebrate in a positive manner without interfering with your lifestyle goals. If you think that your life will become boring if you interrupt a cycle of immediate gratification, challenge yourself to find creative solutions that help you celebrate and meet your lifestyle goals.

Binge Eating

Binge eating means that you consume quantities of food that are definitely more than most people eat over any two-hour period, and you feel that you have lost control and can't stop. Binge eaters often engage in opposite behaviors after bingeing, like taking laxatives, fasting, vomiting, or exercising excessively to "undo" the effect of eating. If this pattern is present at least twice per week for three months, then you may have a problem that needs the help of a psychologist or psychiatrist who specializes in eating disorders. A thorough evaluation of your eating is needed to rule out a more serious problem. Talk with your primary-care physician about the resources available in your community. If you don't know where to start, see the Resources section or Professional Referals. When binge eating is out of control, then your progress toward your goals will likely be negatively affected. Controlling binge eating is a necessary first step in meeting your weight loss and exercise goals.

Strategies for Staying on Track

When practicing patience seems difficult, try some of the strategies listed below:

Practice Waiting in Other Areas

Practicing patience toward attaining your weight-loss and exercise goals will be easier if you practice patience in your life in general. Find ways to exercise patience when you don't want to do so. Purposely take your time. Challenge the notion that you must do *anything* in a big rush. Choose the longest line and reward yourself for being calm and patient. Patience takes practice, so keep at it until you learn this lesson well.

Use Techniques You Know

The skill of mindful focus presented in chapter 5 can help increase your patience. Review your goals, being sure that your short-term goals are reasonable and doable. It's easier to be patient when you focus on small, achievable milestones in front of you.

Know Your Patterns

One of the best tools you have for preparing for times in which you might be vulnerable is to know the specific times, places, and situations in which you are likely to slip. When you are familiar with your vulnerabilities, you can learn to anticipate and plan for them.

Don't Deprive Yourself

Challenge the thought that you are desperate or in dire straits. Be flexible about fulfilling your needs so you don't create a real or imagined state of deprivation. When you give to yourself in healthy ways, you will be giving yourself much more than you ever could by giving in to your need for instant gratification.

Are Unruly Emotions Ruling Your Life?

Emotions are wonderful creations. Without them, you would miss feeling joy, love, and excitement. Neither would you have hurt or frustration to signal you that there is a problem in need of attention. As one of the most common hidden barriers, emotions can become unruly, sometimes sneaking up on you in ways you don't foresee to derail your weight-loss and exercise goals. The focus of this chapter is on how and why emotions interfere with attaining your goals. You will learn how your specific emotion, food, and exercise connections contribute to veering off track. Techniques for managing difficult, uncomfortable emotions related to your food and exercise choices will be introduced. You will also learn to interrupt the negative emotional cycle that keeps you from progressing toward your goals.

What Are Unruly Emotions?

You may or may not be aware of the role your emotions play in eating and exercise. Food provides comfort, leading many people to eat in response to negative emotions, such as sadness or anxiety. You may also eat when there's no strong emotion, but when you feel kind of "blah." Positive emotions may also play a role in your eating and exercise behavior. You may reward yourself with food or give yourself a "break" from exercise as a reward for an achievement or as a celebration. These emotions and reactions are common and can be built into your life in such a way that you can still meet your goals. Unruly emotions are those emotions that affect your food and exercise choices in a manner that is not in your best interest. Being unaware of your emotions and how they affect your food and exercise choices can derail your goals and good health habits.

How Emotions Lead You off Track with Weight Loss

So how *do* emotions affect eating and exercise? This is a complicated question that is still being studied, but in this chapter, you'll learn some important findings from the research. Eating is connected with emotions and past experience. Food can be linked with positive emotions, such as eating with abandon because you're happy or celebrating. You might have learned to reward yourself with food based on childhood experiences in which caregivers gave you sweets as praise for good behavior. Although positive emotions can hijack your goals when you use them to further heighten your moods, especially in times of celebration, more often overeating is connected with negative emotions such as depression, anxiety, loneliness, and boredom.

Thayer (2001) describes one of the most promising answers to the question of how moods are associated with overeating in his book *Calm Energy: How People Regulate Mood with Food and Exercise*. He believes that negative emotions and overeating are related to a condition that he calls *tense tiredness*. Tense tiredness is a state of low energy and increased tension that often accompanies negative emotions. Tense tiredness can be described by that restless sense that you don't like what you are feeling, yet don't feel like doing anything about it. This state is described when someone says, "Sometimes I'm so wound up and tired that I just don't care whether I eat healthy foods." Sweets and junk food cause increases in blood sugar that provide a quick, yet temporary, cure to the negative emotions and the tense tiredness that accompanies them. The relief and increased energy we feel after eating serves to reinforce the value and power of eating as a strategy to cope with emotions. Thayer notes that food becomes like a drug that is used to temporarily relieve negative emotional states. Using food to relieve tension and negative emotions, such as guilt, depression, and frustration, often leads to a cycle of overeating that, in turn, increases negative emotions. Learning to overcome the emotion-food-relief cycle by directly attending to the real problem, that is, your negative emotions, can help you stay on track with your healthy eating goals.

How Emotions Lead You off Track with Exercise

Exercise produces endorphins, which are chemicals inside the body that activate opiate receptors in the brain, making us feel good. Seasoned exercisers say that they can't live without the stress relief and the good feelings that exercise promotes. However, the same phenomenon described for the emotion-food connection is present in the emotion-exercise relationship.

You monitor your energy level throughout the day without even thinking about it. When negative emotions and tense tiredness are present, the motivation required to start your exercise plans decreases. Good intentions to exercise and even well-practiced exercise habits can be interrupted when you give in to tense tiredness.

You may be able to relate to having a day in which you fully intend to exercise, but are derailed by other responsibilities, a last-minute request, or schedule alterations. You arrive at home feeling tense and tired, and you lack the energy necessary to exercise. These feelings make it hard, if not impossible, to meet your goal.

Alternatively, emotions and beliefs connected to those emotions can lead some individuals to exercise more than is generally reasonable. When emotions or tense tiredness hijack your good intentions to exercise or lead you to exercise in a compulsive manner, then you must make an effort to take control of how you handle negative emotions and a general lack of energy.

How Are You Doing Now?

Like many individuals who ask for help with weight loss, you may know without a doubt that emotions derail your weight-loss and exercise goals. You may even label yourself an "emotional eater." On the other hand, you may not be aware of how emotions influence your weight-loss and exercise efforts. Discover some clues by checking off the statements that apply to you.

☐ I often find myself eating "without thinking."

☐ Eating helps me when I'm "blah," depressed, or down.

☐ I reward myself with breaks from exercise and healthy eating.

☐ I downplay the importance of emotions in my eating and exercise behaviors.

☐ I feel a sense of tension or urgency prior to overeating.

☐ I often eat when I'm not hungry.

☐ Most of the time, I feel a need to "just relax" rather than exercise.

☐ I tend to gain or lose weight when I experience stress.

☐ I am often too tired or stressed to exercise.

If you answered no to most or all of these questions, then emotions may not be a primary cause for you getting off track with your weight loss and exercise goals. If several of these questions were answered with a yes, then there is good news: there are specific and scientifically sound ways you can begin to tame the emotions that trip you up and lead you off track.

How Can You Be More Successful?

Before you can develop a solution to any challenge, you need to define the challenge as completely as possible. The more specific you can be about the type of emotion(s) that lead you off track and the situations associated with them, the better you'll be at creating a set of solutions that is right for you. With a little work, you can reap big rewards toward a healthy lifestyle. So, put on your scientist's hat and begin to observe yourself.

Identify the Emotion

Can you easily identify the emotions that are present when you're veering off track with your weight-loss or exercise goals? A sure-fire way to find out which emotions are present at which times is to keep a written record. There is no substitute for the good data that results from daily observation of yourself. Pick a period of time you think you can manage. A week is a good start, but a few days is fine. Place a few index cards in your purse or pocket and begin to observe your behavior. When you catch yourself overeating or choosing to skip exercise, pull out a card and write down the situation and the feeling you have at that moment. You can do so by completing the statement, "I'm feeling _____ right now." If your style is to keep track of what you eat and the fat and calories associated, then simply add the feelings you have in your food diary. You don't have to write a book; just write some quick, short notes. The headings on your paper can include the date, the situation, the feeling, and how you were off track. An example might be finding yourself eating lunch at your desk while reviewing your notes before a meeting. You might find yourself eating more than usual and record that you were feeling so anxious or upset that you didn't prepare more thoroughly. Eating a large lunch and a candy bar might be how you were off track with your goals.

For now, think about the last time you noticed yourself veering from your weight loss and exercise goals. Where were you? What were you doing? Imagine yourself in that situation and remember what you were feeling at that moment. If nothing comes to mind, ask yourself what you were thinking about and see if you connect with a particular emotion. Go ahead and make a guess as to what you might have been feeling. With practice, you will get better at accurately identifying the feeling.

Take Responsibility for Your Emotions

The second step after identifying your emotions is to admit that they belong to you and are a reaction to your internal or external circumstances. When you experience strong emotions, especially negative ones, you may tend to blame others for "making" you feel a certain way. Of course, you are the only one who can determine and change your reactions to events. Taking responsibility for your emotions doesn't mean denying your emotions. It simply means that whatever it is you feel, you "own" it and don't blame others for it. Your partner or spouse may anger you, but he or she is not to blame for your feelings or overeating in response to those feelings.

Learn Two Techniques for Handling Emotions

There are many ways to take control of your emotions. We have grouped a series of techniques into what we call directive and shift-away strategies. Some strategies will work better than others, depending on the type of emotion and situation. Some may not work well for you at all. Try them all to discover which techniques work best for you. At the end of this chapter, there are questions to help you choose whether to use a directive or shift-away strategy.

Directive Strategies

Directive strategies help you focus directly on the feeling, experience it, and do something active to address it. Below are some of our favorite directive strategies.

Find the thought and change it. Emotions are preceded by thoughts, even when you feel as though you aren't thinking anything. A man whose wife died recently identified that he was prone to overeat when he felt sad and lonely when he was home alone. When he began to notice his thoughts, he found he was saying to himself, "I can't tolerate being alone. I will never be able to handle this." However, a review of the facts showed that he *was* tolerating his wife's death, even though it was difficult. Changing your thoughts involves: 1) bringing your thoughts in line with what is realistic and accurate and 2) fully recognizing the strengths and resources you have to handle the emotions and the situation. When he substituted more realistic and resourceful thoughts, such as, "Feeling sad is hard. I am grieving. I can learn to tolerate these feelings," his emotions changed. Telling himself that he could handle his feelings helped Jack feel more confident that his strong feelings would pass.

If finding the thoughts that accompany the emotion is difficult for you, use the index card method to track your thoughts and feelings for a week. For example, when you feel a strong emotion, ask yourself to complete the statement, "When I feel _____ , I'm thinking _____ ." This exercise will help you identify the thoughts associated with your emotions.

Changing your "I can't handle it" thoughts to ones that are self-encouraging will help you change your emotional state and increase your confidence. Your substitute thoughts need to be positive and realistic. Think of how you would like a supportive person to respond to you. A supportive person would probably say that although your task is difficult, you will be able to accomplish it.

Use problem-solving skills. Emotions are often related to problems that need attention, such as chronic loneliness or boredom. They signal the need for action. Creating a problem-solving plan to address the emotion is far more effective than allowing it to continue to interrupt your healthy eating and exercise goals. If you feel loneliness before you begin to over-eat, use the feeling as a cue to make a plan to increase your social activities. Are you bored? Embark on a program to discover what other activities or hobbies would entice you. Are you anxious? Figure out what is causing your anxiety and make a plan to confront it. Resolving more of the difficult, long-standing problems may take time, effort, and possibly professional assistance, but it is extraordinarily more helpful to confront the problem than to allow the emotions to continue to derail your game plan.

Experience the emotion. Another directive method of addressing any feeling is to simply focus on it and allow it to move on. As hard as it is to believe sometimes, the intensity of feelings does pass. To try this technique, the next time you feel like your weight-loss or exercise goals are going off track, identify the emotion. Then, sit down and allow yourself to feel the emotion fully. Notice the physical sensations that you have. Focus your attention directly on the feeling and try to experience it as a wave passing through you.

For a short time, you may feel intense sadness or anxiety. Try to maintain your focus on the feeling, and then let the intensity pass. You will probably be surprised that the emotion has less punch when you experience it. This technique should not be used when you are feeling intense anger, since focusing on anger serves to reinforce and strengthen the angry thoughts. Try one of the problem-solving or shift-away techniques if anger is the negative emotion.

Remind yourself of the game plan. When your emotions become unruly, remind yourself of the game plan. At that critical moment when you are tempted to eat or not exercise in response to emotions, you have the opportunity to choose to pay attention to the feeling or to the larger goal—your good health. Remind yourself of why you want to eat healthy foods and exercise. Picture yourself reaching your goal and envision what it feels like. See yourself attaining and maintaining your weight-loss and exercise goals. If the emotion or the goal is going to win your attention, build a strong case for focusing on the big-picture goal and your future success.

Shift-Away Strategies

Shift-away strategies are those that help you focus on something else, shifting your thoughts away from the emotion.

These strategies are especially helpful in giving you some time to calm yourself before you act on the emotion.

Breathe deeply and relax. Few strategies will decrease a heightened physiological state, such as tension or anxiety, like breathing from your diaphragm and learning to deeply relax your muscles. Deep breathing involves using your diaphragm and breathing slow, deep breaths. To try breathing deeply, place both of your hands at the bottom of your rib cage. Walk your fingers on both sides to the middle and you will find a soft portion of your abdomen. Place one of your hands over this spot. Now, breathe naturally, but slowly and deeply. If you are breathing using your diaphragm, your hand will move up and down when you breathe. When you are sure you are breathing from your diaphragm, take ten slow, deep breaths, making the exhalations a little longer than the inhalations. After this time-out, you may be better able to evaluate your situation more objectively.

For a quick relaxation exercise, sit or lie down, close your eyes, and take ten slow, deep breaths. Focus your mental energy on the tension that may be present in your body. Imagine a wave of warm, soothing relaxation beginning at your head and slowly moving over your head, neck, shoulders, arms, torso, legs, and feet. As you breathe, allow the tension to leave your body. Notice that your muscles might feel warm, heavy, or tingling as they relax. Do a second sweep of the warm wave, imagining it beginning at the top of your head and moving slowly down and through your body. Try these techniques when you begin to feel overwhelmed. Relaxing for a few minutes can help you feel refreshed and able to focus on your healthy eating and exercise goals. These techniques go a long way to resolve the feeling of tense tiredness without overeating.

Try Self-Soothing. Everyone has activities that give them a sense of comfort and soothe their emotions. Unfortunately, many of us are taught to soothe negative emotions with food.

Alternative examples of self-soothing strategies are taking a walk, soaking in a warm bath, lighting candles, writing in a journal, or making crafts. Search your environment for soothing elements that relate to your senses. Identify sights, smells, textures, and sounds that help you feel better. These strategies can be as simple as putting on some scented lotion. Physical exercise is a great way to interrupt negative emotions. Take a brisk walk around your neighborhood or perform some stretching exercises at home to give you a break from the emotion. You might also decide to do something productive you've been putting off. Perform yoga, meditate, or pray. Find the right self-soothing strategies to help lessen your negative emotion and state of tense tiredness.

Engage in the opposite emotion. Another way to shift away from the emotion that is bothering you is to engage in an activity that will help you experience the opposite emotion. If you are depressed and sad, think of a pleasurable activity and begin to do that. Act as if you are happy. If you're frustrated and angry, find an activity that helps you be nice to someone. Don't make the mistake of believing you will lose something by letting go of anger. The bigger mistake is to hold on to it and lose focus on what you really want in life. If you are feeling anxious, do something that makes you feel calm. Act like you don't have a worry in the world. Do you feel as though you have no energy? Do something that refreshes you and act like you have a large energy reserve. Acting the opposite of how you feel may seem awkward and fake at first. Hang in there. Engaging in the opposite emotion can help you shift away from the negative emotions and tense tiredness you feel and help you take control.

Should I Use a Shift-Away or Directive Strategy?

When to use a shift-away or directive strategy will be based on your judgment and experience. There is no one right way to manage your unruly emotions. Remember that you need to practice these strategies for them to be effective. Your unruly emotions won't go down without a fight. To help you choose which type of strategy to use, we offer the following questions.

If you answer "yes" to the following questions, a shift-away strategy may be timely:

1. Does this feeling feel "too hot" right now?

2. If you don't calm down quickly, do you think you will act impulsively?

3. Is this a situation you just need to get through, knowing it isn't likely to happen again soon?

If you answer "yes" to the following questions, a directive strategy may be timely:

1. Is there likely an underlying problem that I am avoiding?

2. Is this a good time for me to learn to confront and gain control over this type of emotion?

3. Do I think this emotion is likely to come back and continue to interfere with my game plan?

Have an Emotional-Trigger Plan

You now know how emotions can interrupt your good intentions, plans, and determination to lose weight and exercise. You have identified some of your high-risk situations and have learned strategies to handle these emotions. You can help yourself further if you make an emotional-trigger plan. An emotional-trigger plan alerts you to when and how your emotions are usurping your objectivity and undermining your progress, and it includes strategies you personally have found effective.

To begin making your emotional-trigger plan, review the information you've compiled from this chapter. List the top five situations in which you are most likely to abandon healthy eating and exercise. List the top five physical cues that remind you of these times, such as tired eyes, a knot in your stomach, or a headache. List the top five feelings that are likely to be a part of these situations. Then, list the top five thoughts that seem to precede or be associated with these feelings. (An example is that feeling frustrated might be accompanied by the thought, "My boss never understands my situation.") When you're finished, list the directive or shift-away strategies that have been helpful to you in these situations. Look over the emotional-trigger plan several times a day for the first few weeks until you've learned it well. Review and update the plan thereafter on a regular basis. With your emotional-trigger plan in hand and your understanding of how to manage unruly emotions, you are one step closer to realizing your goals.

Why Are You Getting off Track?

If the exercises presented for this solution don't seem to help you identify and change the way your emotions impact your lifestyle behaviors, consider whether one of these reasons is part of the difficulty.

You Need the Unruly Emotion

Sometimes the inability to change unruly emotions is due to the fact that the emotion serves some larger purpose in your life, and effectively handling that emotion means that other aspects of your life will change. Perhaps a feeling of constant frustration helps you feel productive. Feelings of anger may be a front for avoiding feeling down or hurt. Perhaps feeling overwhelmed on a constant basis helps you gain assistance from others. Most of the time, the functions unruly emotions serve aren't worth it, but thinking about changing them initially may be difficult. These realizations can be hard to discern and you may need professional assistance to overcome them if they are long-standing patterns. Ask yourself what possible purpose the unruly emotion has in your life and then evaluate whether it is really worth experiencing on a consistent basis.

You Are Ambivalent about Change

The persistence of your unruly emotions may be an expression of your ambivalence about change. When you directly address the reasons you are veering off track from your healthy eating and exercise goals, you face the probability of change. Any change is scary, and ambivalence is a natural part of the process. Review your Pro-Con Balance Sheet from chapter 2 to remind yourself of your reasons for wanting to change. Additionally, find ways to reinforce the positive aspects of the lifestyle changes you are making.

Your Unruly Emotions Are a More Serious Problem

Sometimes unruly emotions are indicators of more serious psychiatric conditions, such as depression or anxiety. Seek professional help for an expert opinion about whether you have more serious difficulties with depression or anxiety (See Professional Referrals in Resources). After receiving treatment, you will likely be better able to implement the solutions in this book.

Strategies for Staying on Track

The following are strategies for staying on track with handling unruly emotions.

Add Emotions to Your Goals and Game Plan

Incorporate your learning about managing emotions into your goals and game-plan strategies. Your goal might address the most challenging situations you have with managing emotions. Adopt some of the strategies in this chapter into your daily game-plan strategies to further your learning and progress toward your goals.

Notice the Purpose of the Emotion

If your emotions are serving a purpose in your life that is not productive or helpful, identify the reasons and address them directly. For example, if you find that anger is hiding other emotions, such as depression or hurt, begin to address the real feelings. If you are honest about what you are feeling and deal directly with the situation, you will be better able to act in your best interest.

Schedule Practice Time

Part of implementing the solutions in this chapter may involve scheduling time to practice the interventions suggested. Adding practice to your schedule can help.

In this chapter, you've learned several techniques to manage unruly emotions, a very common difficulty that may have led you off track in the past. Mastering this hidden barrier will go a long way toward helping you achieve your weight-loss and exercise goals.

How Do You Treat Your Mistakes?

One of the greatest challenges in your exercise and weight-loss plan is to react effectively when you make a mistake. The mistake might be a late-night snack, putting off exercise for another day, or having an extra dessert. These mistakes can simply be minor slips, with no significant impact on your overall game plan. However, depending on how you respond, slips can turn into setbacks, and become a hidden barrier. In this chapter, we will use the terms mistake, slip, and getting off track interchangeably, referring to any action that is counter to your exercise and weight-loss goals.

What Is Treating Your Mistakes as Useful?

This chapter is devoted to helping you manage your slips and setbacks in the most effective and efficient means possible.

Toward that goal, you will learn to not just "get by" your mistakes, but to understand them and respond in a way that actually helps your change efforts. No one likes to make mistakes. But if you are going to make them, then you'll need to know how to think and react most effectively.

Treating your mistakes as useful is critical because of two important rules for achieving your goals:

Rule #1: You are going to have mistakes and slips along the way.

Rule #2: It is a mistake to argue against Rule #1.

Why shouldn't you expect yourself to make a plan, set it in action, and stick to it without fail? It certainly sounds like an appropriate and positive outlook. The fact is that most people just don't proceed through the process of making change in an even and linear fashion. Rather, research reveals that a more typical process is one where people have slips and setbacks. In their stages of change model discussed in chapter 2, Prochaska and DiClemente visualized this process as a "spiral of change," where people make progress toward their goals, then slip back to earlier habits before moving on again.

By viewing your change efforts on a spiral, you can expect yourself to achieve your goals *while* you make mistakes. You won't be surprised when you do slip and have an extra dessert or if you don't exercise as scheduled. As you consider mistakes to be a part of the process, you won't be as susceptible to strong emotional reactions, such as anger, disgust, or disappointment. These emotions can become difficult to manage and can direct your focus away from your healthy goals. By expecting mistakes to be part of the process, you can keep a more calm and objective mind-set as you consider what to do following a mistake.

Your view of mistakes as useful will also help prepare you for how to deal with them. With the appropriate expectations, a calm demeanor, and thoughtful consideration about how best to respond, you will be better prepared to address the mistake and get yourself back on track. Knowing that you can and will be able to deal with your mistakes is also helpful with maintaining the changes over the long run. Slips and setbacks can become discouraging. If you believe that you know how to deal with them, you will be less likely to get discouraged or demoralized.

Another reason why mistakes are important to achieving your goals is that no game plan will be perfect right off the bat. You will need to learn along the way that your mistakes are a wonderful source of feedback about what you may need to do differently. If you are open and curious, your mistakes will reveal things you forgot to consider in your game plan, such as external factors that interfere with your scheduled exercise, emotional reactions that will need special attention, or times when you need extra help with your focus. Without a productive attitude toward mistakes, many game plans don't get the modifications necessary to lead to successful change.

Finally, treating your mistakes as useful requires that you treat yourself well. You must recognize that you're only human. Getting off track doesn't mean that you have to punish yourself. Rather, you can respond with your best interest in mind. Think about how such an attitude can relate to all the pursuits and goals in your life. No matter what you're trying to accomplish, a supportive and helpful approach will make the work more enjoyable and likely more successful.

How Are You Doing Now?

In an effort to get an accurate appraisal of how you currently respond to your mistakes, check off the statements that describe you:

☐ I try not to think about the things I do that get me off track.

☐ When I slip from my game plan, I have a strong emotional reaction.

☐ I repeat the same mistakes but don't understand why.

☐ Reflecting on my mistakes usually makes me feel worse.

☐ It really bothers me if others know when I have slipped from my plans.

If the majority of these statements describe you, your reactions to mistakes may be playing an important role in achieving your goals. Read and follow the steps below to gain a better understanding of how you respond to your mistakes.

Step 1: Find examples of when you were off track from your game plan

Search your memory for when you made a mistake or slip with your exercise or weight-loss game plan. It can be a minor slip that had no significant consequences or a setback in which you got away from your game plan for a week. The more recent the example, the better, as you will be trying to recall a number of details about what occurred.

Step 2: Identify your thoughts and feelings when you recognized the mistake

How you think about the situation, your actions, the change process, and yourself will have an impact on your reaction. You will also be having some kind of feeling or emotion related to what happened. And you'll have some thoughts about those feelings. The mind is a busy place, but don't worry. With practice, you will be able to zero in on the thoughts and feelings that are having the most influence on your reaction. Use the following questions to help you:

1. What was your immediate feeling when you first realized you had slipped?

2. Was there another feeling that followed your immediate emotional response?

3. What were the immediate thoughts that went through your mind when you realized you made the mistake?

4. Did you make any quick conclusions about yourself, your character, or your ability to successfully change habits?

Step 3: Identify what you actually did in response to the mistake

The bottom line with your reaction to mistakes is what comes of it. How will it impact you and your goals? In order to know this impact, you must first be able to clearly identify your actions following the mistake. Did you think of things you could do differently next time, quickly move on to something else, or somehow punish yourself? To help you identify your actions following a mistake, consider the following suggestions:

1. Be concrete and specific. What did you do, where did you go?

2. Be aware that not doing anything is a reaction. Whatever you did or didn't do should be noted.

3. Be aware of your later reactions. You will likely have an immediate response to your realization of a slip, but will also have reactions later, which should be noted. You may have later reactions to the original mistake or even reactions to your reactions (such as, "I'm so angry that I just dismissed that slip last night").

4. Don't analyze or judge yet. This step is about accurately and objectively becoming aware of what is happening when you make mistakes.

Your reactions to getting off track often become automatic and are not easily identified. As part of the previous self-assessment steps, you are encouraged to record your responses to past and present mistakes. Create a "Reactions to Mistakes Log" by drawing four vertical columns on a sheet of paper. The column headings will be, "The Mistake I Made," "Emotional Reaction," "Automatic Thoughts," and "What I Did Next." Fill in across the columns for each mistake. Later in the chapter you will learn about effective strategies for responding to slips and setbacks. You will then want to add a fifth column to your log, entitled "My New Effective Response."

How Can You Be More Successful?

This section will describe the critical components of treating your mistakes as useful and offer specific strategies to help you integrate them into your change efforts.

Make Your Expectations Realistic

You now know, and have likely known for a long time, that mistakes are part of the game. You may have shared this piece of wisdom with your children or friends. However, sometimes saying it to yourself is another story. You need to realistically estimate how likely you are to have a slip from your game plan. The exact number doesn't matter. What is important is that you recognize the possibility of mistakes and won't be shocked when they occur. Don't be too easy on yourself and anticipate plenty of slips. You want to balance the reality that we all make mistakes with the need to expect yourself to stick to your game plan.

Anticipate High-Risk Situations

There are going to be situations and conditions where you have a higher risk of getting off track with your game plan. This is another opportunity for you to anticipate well and not let yourself be surprised by difficult situations. Think about your high-risk situations and when you have gotten off track in the past. Are there certain times of the day? Are slips more likely when you are tired or have low energy? Are certain social situations a factor? Being aware of these times will help you anticipate and plan, or at least recover quickly if you do have a momentary slip.

Catch and Return to Your Game Plan

An important strategy for dealing with your mistakes will likely be a quick "catch and return" technique. With this strategy, you recognize that you are off track from your game plan and quickly get yourself back on track. When you become aware of the mistake, you want to take responsibility for what you did, recognize that it wasn't what you wanted to do, and then calmly direct yourself back to the game plan. This redirection may involve some immediate action (such as putting the snack away or getting up from the table) or planning for what you will do (for example, exercise that evening, buy fruit on the way home). The following strategies will help you successfully catch your mistakes and return to the game plan.

Practice Responsibility for Your Reaction

Every moment after a slip is an opportunity to responsibly and thoughtfully decide what you need to do next. Work on not letting yourself off the hook or avoiding this responsibility. Envision how you will catch the mistakes and what you will say to yourself, and responsibly carry out your plan.

Review the chapter on practicing the skill of responsibility for a more in-depth discussion.

Allow Only Productive Thinking

By allowing only the thinking that will be helpful, you will be more likely to stop going over the mistake in your mind without any specific purpose, replaying the visual images of what you did, or using negative, discouraging self-talk. Practice a new connection between making a mistake and only thinking about it if it will be of help to you.

Use Laughter and Lightness

Perspective is a very helpful tool in dealing with mistakes. When you have the right perspective, you realize that mistakes aren't the end of the world. Better yet, you can laugh at what you did. You messed up, and will probably do something like it again. You . . . you . . . you . . . human! Join the club.

Tell a Friend about Your Mistake

There is a common tendency to want to keep mistakes, slips, and difficulties a secret. This strengthens the idea that they should be avoided and not be seen in the light of day. Why not do the opposite? Laugh with a trusted friend about what you did. Tell them not to feel bad for you or offer advice. It's not that big of a deal and you know what to do differently. You just want to "out" the mistake so you can catch it quickly and effortlessly in the future.

Do Something Concrete toward Your Goal

Find something to do toward your exercise and weight-loss goal that is concrete and action-oriented. Eat a piece of fruit, write out your specific dinner menu for the evening, walk two flights of stairs, or do ten push-ups. Do something, anything, that helps you recall your reasons for doing this work and that you can do it. There is nothing better than concrete actions to set you back on track.

Talk to Yourself Like a Good Coach

Use your self-talk to guide you in catching the mistake and calmly redirecting yourself back on track. Like a good coach, remind yourself of your resiliency and strength to squarely address your mistakes. Coach yourself to relax, keep the mistake in perspective, stay in a helpful mind-set, and simply get back to what you know is best for you.

Stop and Learn from Your Mistakes

With each slip or setback, you have the opportunity to learn and improve your change efforts. Remember that we learn best in a calm, objective, and noncritical environment. You also want to make sure your focus is helpful and productive. Simply rehashing what happened is likely to make you feel worse.

As you review the mistake, ask yourself, "What may have motivated me to do that?" What really happened there?" or "What could I have done differently?" What else should you be learning or looking for? It will be helpful to have some ideas of the things that could be useful to learn about. Use the following areas to help guide your questions and reflections of when you got off track.

Assess Your Reactions

How do you know how you react to mistakes? Are you responding in a productive or counterproductive style? The only way to really know is to make mistakes and reflect on how you responded in that situation. As you experienced in the self-assessment section, your mistakes give you the opportunity to ask about your thoughts, feelings, and subsequent reactions.

Explore Other Hidden Barriers

Many of the chapters in this book are designed to help you understand and plan for the challenges to staying on track. Whether it is managing emotions, staying focused, or being ready for change, your particular challenges reveal themselves through your mistakes. Look at what happened when you got off track as a guide to help you identify the issues in this book that will be most relevant for you.

Make Adjustments

Your initial game plan for losing weight and exercising will likely need to be adjusted as you gain experience in using it. Use your mistakes to reveal and guide what needs to change. Is your game plan accounting for such issues as the time it takes to exercise, the best time for your snacks, or how often you need reminders?

When to "Stop and Learn" Rather Than "Catch and Return"

How do you know whether to stop and learn from your mistake, rather than catch it and quickly return to the game plan? The answer is a judgment on your part. Often, the most efficient thing is to simply catch the mistake and jump right back on track. However, there are times when it may be smart to stop and really try to learn something valuable. Reflecting on what you did and learning from it may be warranted if the following apply: the mistake is repetitive and showing no decrease in how often it occurs; you don't understand why the mistake is happening; the mistake is badly getting you off track or leading to larger setbacks; or the "catch and return" strategy isn't working.

Practice a Positive Attitude about Mistakes

The mistakes you make in your weight-loss and exercise efforts may reveal how you think about making mistakes in other areas of your life. You have the opportunity here to check in with your overall outlook on mistakes. Do you value mistakes? Do you see them as something to hide from others? You are encouraged to view your mistakes as: an unavoidable part of life; opportunities to learn and to grow; something that happens to everyone; part of being likeable and approachable; not a reflection of your value or worth as a person; and part of an open and nondefensive style.

For some, these beliefs may seem normal and natural. However, you may feel like these ideas sound good but don't really apply to you. Try them on and practice acting "as if" you believe this way. Your old beliefs are not set in stone, and this new way of looking at mistakes may grow on you.

Why Are You Getting off Track?

Having thought about what you can do to successfully manage your mistakes, you will also want to be aware of how you react to mistakes that may get you off track. This section discusses a number of reactions that people have that cause their mistakes to be unproductive and often destructive to achieving their goals.

You Become Angry with Yourself

One common reaction to getting off track with your exercise or weight-loss plan is to get angry with yourself. An immediate reaction of frustration would seem to be under-standable when you recognize that you have done something counter to your goals. However, a moment of frustration can quickly escalate into anger toward yourself. Often this anger is not expressed outwardly but takes place in the privacy of your thoughts and feelings. If you're getting angry with yourself when you make a mistake, you may: use harsh, critical, judg-mental words to describe yourself; have unrealistic, demand-ing, or perfectionistic expectations of yourself; believe that all mistakes deserve to be punished; view anger as motivating and helpful, or use anger to avoid feeling down or bad about yourself.

Rather than being motivating or helpful, anger toward yourself usually makes working on your goals much more aversive or difficult. If you're like most people, you will have difficulty sustaining any project in which you are subject to angry reactions. You'll probably end up developing a hidden agenda of wanting to get away from this anger and pressure.

You Feel Guilty and Bad about Yourself

Feeling guilty and bad about yourself may be your reac-tion to getting off track. The bad feelings, which can be very intense, stem from how you think about yourself and what you have done. Do you think of your mistakes as "bad" things that never should have been allowed to happen? How do you think about yourself when you don't exercise or eat well, as you wanted to? Some people will think of the mistake as clear evi-dence of their ineptness, laziness, or not being a good person.

If you are reacting to your mistakes by feeling very bad or guilty, you may be exaggerating the consequences or impor-tance of the mistake, making global conclusions about your character and worth as a person, or thinking of yourself as inferior or somehow inadequate. As with the anger reaction, feeling excessively bad or guilty can easily make your efforts too aversive. Feeling bad about your mistakes can make it too costly for you to pursue your goals. Similar to the anger response, you may develop an agenda to protect yourself from having these bad and guilty feelings and drop the goal.

You Dismiss the Mistake

Another response to slipping up is to view the mistake in such a way that it no longer bothers you. With a quick spin of your reasoning, you can take the mistake off your plate so that you don't have to deal with what happened. One way you may do this is to justify or rationalize what you did. You might tell yourself that you deserved the extra helping because you were particularly stressed or by saying that the slip wasn't a problem since you did some exercise that day. Another strategy for dismissing the mistake is to minimize the consequences.

A dismissal of the mistake allows you to quickly avoid the mistake and any uncomfortable feelings or reactions that may follow. Dismissing the mistake should not be confused with deciding that the mistake was not significant and that you should simply move on. In the latter, there is a judgment about the mistake and how best to respond. Dismissing the mistake is done to quickly distance yourself and avoid addressing the slip altogether. If you react to your mistakes by dismissing them, you may be: avoiding important feedback about your difficulties and weaknesses, reinforcing a habit of seeing things as you would prefer them to be, protecting yourself against anticipated criticism and judgment, or practicing an old habit of not holding yourself responsible.

You Distract Yourself

Similar to dismissing the mistake, distracting yourself is typically an impulsive move to simply make the mistake "go away." Following a moment of awareness that you haven't exercised like you intended or eaten as planned, you may distract yourself by quickly turning your mind back to work, responsibilities at home, or other activities on your agenda. Others will distract themselves with television as a means to occupy their mind. Distraction of any type robs you of the opportunity to reflect and mindfully choose what would be in your best interest. If you are responding to your mistakes by distracting yourself, you may have: difficulty focusing on your areas of weakness; a low tolerance for frustration; difficulty with your focus and responsibility skills; or the idea that addressing mistakes is too aversive or uncomfortable.

You Tell Yourself the Whole Game Plan Is Shot

Have you ever had a slip with your eating or exercise plan and reacted with an extreme, all-or-nothing thought that the game plan is now ruined? If so, you may be viewing your game plan as something that must be adhered to in an absolute fashion, as if any deviation from it is like a fall from grace. With this all-or-nothing perspective, mistakes can quickly lead to the conclusion that you have "blown it," and you may as well go ahead and eat the rest of the cake or skip out on exercise altogether. If you are responding to a mistake with a belief that your whole game plan is ruined, perhaps you: expect that the game plan should be followed in a perfect and absolute manner; view any mistake as a complete failure or collapse of the game plan; fail to recognize your ability or responsibility to deal directly with the mistake; or find yourself having to recover from larger and more frequent setbacks.

It's quite likely that you identified with more than one of these reactions. Many people may initially react negatively toward themselves, and then look to resolve that discomfort by distracting themselves or dismissing what happened. For example, anger or guilt toward yourself can be decreased by quickly moving to another activity or numbing out in front of the television. Once you've identified these habits, you can directly challenge them and get yourself back to treating your mistakes as necessary and useful.

Strategies for Staying on Track

You are encouraged to experiment with each of the following strategies for staying on track. Remember, many of them require practice and repetition for lasting effectiveness.

Manage the Negative Emotions

The reactions to mistakes that lead you to get off track often begin with an unruly, uncomfortable emotion. Whether it is embarrassment, guilt, disappointment, or anger, your emotions need to be identified and effectively managed. Chapter 7 offers specific strategies and tools to help you manage these emotions and keep yourself on track.

Challenge Your Old Beliefs about Mistakes

Throughout your lifetime, you have collected thoughts, beliefs, and assumptions about what it means to make mistakes. You have ideas about what certain mistakes mean about you as a person, the goal you are working on, how you are supposed to react to yourself, and how others may think of you. These beliefs can strongly influence how you feel about the mistake and what will come of the mistake. Write down your beliefs and examine them carefully. Use your adult logic, wisdom, and experience to identify and challenge those beliefs that you don't think are accurate or helpful. They may have made sense at an earlier time in your life, but may no longer be reasonable given how you want to live today.

Make Good Judgments about How Bad You Should Feel

You don't get to decide how bad to feel, do you? Actually, yes. Feeling bad about yourself is largely determined by your conclusions of how bad what you did really was and what you conclude about yourself based on the mistake. Check to see if you are exaggerating the importance of the mistake. Also, look to see if you are making global, far-reaching conclusions about your character, value, and worth. If you're going to feel bad about what you did, make sure that the intensity of the feelings is proportional to what you did and the importance of the mistake.

Catch and Stop Discouraging and Abusive Talk

It's common to talk to yourself in a way that you would never talk to anyone else. Talking to yourself in a harsh, overly critical manner just brings you down and makes it harder to bounce back after a mistake. Try to yell "stop" in your head to disrupt the negative self-talk. Recognize that the talk is not helpful or deserved. Another strategy is to jump back into a productive activity after getting off track. It's hard to continue the abusive thinking when you are acting in a positive manner.

Who's Supporting You?

Throughout this book, you have been learning new skills and developing a game plan to achieve your weight loss and exercise goals. How well you will stay on track depends in part on the environment you create for this work. As with a new business, young child, or even a small plant, certain conditions are necessary for growth and success to occur. The degree of support you receive from yourself and others can be a hidden barrier to your success. This chapter focuses on creating an environment in which you can develop solutions for lasting change.

What Is a Supportive Environment?

A supportive environment is one that promotes the use of effective thinking and actions that help you reach your healthy goals. In addition, a supportive environment increases the likelihood that you will use effective thinking and actions repeatedly. By promoting the use of your best resources, the environment plays a critical role in turning what you know you should do into lasting habits.

The supportive environment is largely made up of reactions to your eating and exercise behavior. Supportive reactions include praise and compliments when you stick to your game plan and overcome challenging moments without getting off track. Hearing "Way to go!" or "Fantastic" usually feels great and makes you want to do it again. Support also includes words of encouragement and understanding when you do get off track. When you get reactions like, "That was a really hard situation" and "Okay, that was just one slip," you aren't as likely to blow the mistake out of proportion or get down on yourself. Harsh, angry, or demeaning reactions only make the work more difficult.

The most effective support mixes praise and understanding with encouragement to stick to the work and keep plugging away. "It's not easy, but you can do it!" conveys understanding and support with a push to not let up on the hard work. The underlying belief to this support is, "I deserve to be treated very well as I get the push I need." A comforting response that also encourages you to drop the challenge isn't the kind of support you need. For example, "You look stressed, let me get you some cake," isn't going to get you where you want to go.

Where do these supportive reactions come from? Your supportive environment largely includes people around you who positively influence your eating and exercise behaviors. These people may be family members, friends, people at a gym, or coworkers. As you will learn in this chapter, whom you choose to get support from and how you choose to get that support are important components of successfully creating a supportive environment.

Where else do you get reactions to your eating and exercise behavior? If you counted all the reactions you receive, you likely would find that most of them come from yourself. You are constantly reacting to what you do. Whether it is with a positive comment, a critical one, or more of an emotional reaction, your own reactions make up a big part of the world in which you operate. For this reason, support from yourself will be included as a critical part of creating your supportive environment.

There are a number of important reasons for why creating a supportive environment for your work is so important. First, having a supportive environment will help reinforce your new habits and increase the likelihood of doing them again. It also makes pursuing your goals a much more enjoyable thing to do. You need and deserve a positive and encouraging atmosphere as you pursue your weight loss and exercise goals. This chapter will help you develop that supportive environment, inside and out.

How Are You Doing Now?

An honest and accurate picture of your current supportive environment will be necessary. As always, an accurate understanding of yourself allows you to identify what you are doing well and what specific areas will need further attention. Your internal environment may be quite different than your outside environment and will be evaluated separately.

The first assessment focuses on the private environment that you provide within your own mind. Read the following statements and mark the ones that describe you:

☐ I am quick to get angry at and critical of myself.

☐ I often use anger to motivate myself.

☐ I think praising myself is unnecessary.

☐ Talking to myself with supportive statements seems a little embarrassing.

☐ I think of being supportive as something to do for others, not for myself.

If most of these statements describe you, then you probably can benefit from developing a more supportive style of responding to yourself. Now, look at the support you are getting from others. Again, read the following statements and check off the ones that describe you:

☐ Usually no one knows when I get off track with my game plan.

☐ I don't tell friends or family that I'm trying to be healthier.

☐ I don't tell people how I want to be supported.

☐ I believe that a close family member really would prefer that I not change.

☐ I feel like I have to do things completely on my own.

☐ When I do get encouragement from others, I tend to discount it.

If you agreed with most of these statements, it is quite possible that you will be able to increase the support you get from others. In addition, specific relationships may need to be further evaluated to better understand their impact on your goals.

How Can You Be More Successful?

It's easy to recognize the wisdom of being supportive to yourself and getting it from others. However, creating a supportive environment requires learned skills that may not come so easily. How we have come to treat ourselves and how we expect to be treated by others develops from a young age. Ideally, you grew up in a very supportive, encouraging environment where you learned to treat yourself and others in kind. If you are one of the many people who did not grow up in such an environment, you will need to develop these skills as an adult.

Be Supportive When You Succeed

How do you react when you follow your game plan, overcome tempting eating situations, or exercise when you would rather not? It's important that you react in a manner that encourages and reinforces what you did. One way to do so is to recognize the importance of what you did and feel proud. Shout "Way to go!" and talk as if you were a great coach rooting his or her players on. Think about what you'd really like to hear. Successful moments should also be used as hard evidence that you have the skills and abilities to be successful. If you did it once, you can expect yourself and push yourself to do it again. If you didn't grow up hearing this positive talk, you may be cynical, find it silly, or dismiss it because it feels awkward. Do it anyhow. Positive reinforcement is very important for building good habits and is not reserved just for children.

Be Even More Supportive When You Aren't Successful

"I can be my own worst enemy." This phrase can be especially relevant to how you react to slips. As discussed in chapter 8, How Do You Treat Your Mistakes?, it is important to recognize that slips will happen and that the key is to respond to them effectively. A supportive environment involves acknowledging that you will slip at times, stopping any anger or critical reaction, talking to yourself using encouraging statements, and directing yourself back on track. Examples of such statements include, "Okay, that wasn't pretty, but I'm back on track now" or "Wow, I blew it that time, but I know I have what it takes to hang in there."

Ask the Right People for Support

As you work on giving yourself support, you'll also want to get it from others. Getting support from others is a skill and it begins with making good choices about whom to ask for support. You may be frustrated with the lack of support you're getting from the people in your life. But are you taking responsibility for your choices about whom to ask? Look for people who seem genuinely interested in your welfare and can put aside their needs and attend to yours. Often, you will find that people whom you have supported will be eager to return the favor. If they aren't willing, you may want to evaluate how mutually respectful and collaborative the friendship is.

Do you assume that support and encouragement are part of every relationship? If you do, you're likely to get frustrated with others and simply stop sharing. Giving support is a skill, and the fact is that some people are more skilled and ready to give it than others. Rather than get caught up in trying to get it from a family member or friend who seems disinterested or unwilling, make smart choices and look to someone who is more likely to give you the support you need.

Know What You Need

What acts of support would be most helpful to you? Don't get frustrated if you don't have an immediate answer to this question. Many people don't have a specific awareness of what they need from others. You may find you need words of praise and compliments. You might need encouragement and reminders that you can meet your goals. You may really need support when you have gotten off track and need reassurance and a push to get right back to your game plan. Another kind of support is more instrumental and focuses on helping you implement your game plan. You may need advice on what to eat or how to exercise. With a busy schedule, you may need support in the form of someone helping you readjust your responsibilities. You can't expect others to meet your needs if you don't know what they are.

Teach Others What You Need

How do the people in your life know that you need support and encouragement? Many people make the mistake of assuming that others should know what they need. In fact, teaching people what you need is a critical skill in many areas of a relationship, such as romance, sex, and conflict. It will take a moment of feeling vulnerable, but it's important to let others know when and what kind of support you need.

Tell the person directly what you need. For example, you may say, "I would really appreciate it if you wouldn't suggest we get dessert after each meal" or "I know I don't usually ask, but I'd love a 'way to go' when you see me exercising." You can also practice this directness by asking others what kind of support they want from you. Examples include, "What do you need from me right now?" and "Please tell me how I can be there for you in the future." The person you have chosen may not be accustomed to you directly talking about needing support, so be patient. It will probably take both of you time and repeated talks to get used to your new expectations.

Address Conflicts with Others

A supportive environment also requires not having influences that interfere with your success. These influences can involve people who aren't supportive of your change efforts, and people who do want you to change but express themselves in an unsupportive way. Both groups can create conflicts that need to be addressed.

Unfortunately, there may be someone in your life who doesn't want you to be successful in your weight-loss and exercise efforts. They may directly state their opposition to your goals, with overt threats or critical statements. Some may take a more indirect route and encourage you to get off track by encouraging a "harmless" detour from your game plan or making subtler discouraging comments.

Before you can effectively deal with such individuals, it's important to have some understanding of why they are acting as they are. Most people will oppose another person's growth if the change seems to represent a threat to them. How could your losing weight and being fit be threatening to someone else? Think hard about this other person. If you got healthier and happier, would you be less interested in them and more attracted to others? Might you begin new, healthier relationships? Would you find new activities and have less interest in the old ways of having fun that you shared? Could they feel less control in the relationship as you get more effective in your life? Some of their concerns may be very real and others may simply be a misperception on their part. In either case, you want to learn what your healthier lifestyle means to them.

So what do you do about someone who seems to be opposing the healthy changes in your life? The answer will depend on the person, their importance in your life, and your understanding of why they seem to take that position. If you believe that the person would be willing and open to discuss your concerns, you may want to directly bring up the issue and teach them more about what you need from them. If they are not a significant presence in your life and you don't think they would be willing to change, you may want to distance yourself from the relationship. They were probably not as good a friend as you thought.

If the person is your partner, it will be important for you to address their opposition to your change efforts. Look to understand what your change means for them and try to talk openly about how each of you is seeing the problem. If there are significant anger, power, and control issues, it may be valuable to get help from a mental-health professional or some other third party. If it isn't addressed directly, there is a chance that you will drop your goals as a way of diffusing the conflict.

Some people want to see you succeed, but act in an unsupportive manner. For example, they may get angry with you, use sarcastic humor, or lecture you in an effort to move you toward your goals. While their intent may be to help, it is very hard to see past their irritating and sometimes hurtful ways. Unfortunately, some people are very unskilled at being supportive. If you think they may be open to feedback, teach them what you need. If they seem unwilling to learn or change what they are doing, you may have to look elsewhere for support.

Sarah's Story

Sarah is a forty-three-year-old mother of two. She is busy in her roles as mother, nurse, and wife. Sarah has been described as very caring and supportive toward her husband, children, and friends. Her past attempts at exercising and weight loss have been successful in the short term, but her gains typically fade after three or four months.

As Sarah explored the possible reasons for her lack of long-term success, she recognized something interesting about the supportive environment that she created. Simply, there wasn't much of one. She was very organized about her eating and exercise game plan and viewed her work as a matter-of-fact list of tasks to be done on her own. Positive emotion or encouragement was not thought of as relevant, as she saw her game plan as tasks she was "just supposed to do."

In the early stages Sarah did not need encouragement, as her drive and focus were enough to keep her on track. However, over time her motivation would wane and she would become increasingly frustrated with her slips. She didn't look for an emotional lift or support to help her through these times. Eventually, she would drop her goals as a way to avoid the frustration with herself.

Sarah recognized that she was very focused on being supportive of others, but didn't see herself as needing it. Upon assessing her own supportive environment, she saw that she was really quite cold and unsupportive to herself and would never let others think that she needed encouragement. When she talked about this insight to her husband, he said, "Oh, I've always known that. You're the rock." Once she taught him that she would like to have more emotional support for her goals, he was quite willing to give back to her. As she got more support from others, Sarah slowly changed the matter-of-fact way she spoke to herself. She felt good about challenging this barrier to her weight-loss efforts.

Why Are You Getting off Track?

Armed with strategies for successfully creating a supportive environment, you will also want to keep an eye on what gets you off track from this solution. Consider the following issues that get people off track and watch out for those that best apply to you.

Just Not in the Habit

Many people instinctively know to encourage and praise little children. However, you may not think of yourself or other adults as needing praise. Or you may believe it is important but don't really practice creating support for your efforts.

Getting back on track will require conscious effort to see the need for support and do what is necessary to get it.

Fear of Going Too Far

Some people avoid support and encouragement because they associate it with negative qualities they want to avoid. As an example, you may see praising yourself as bragging or being egotistical. Or you may see asking for encouragement as being needy and a burden. You don't want to be associated with these negative qualities, so you avoid asking for the support you need. But how realistic are your assumptions? Check for unrealistic fears and possible exaggerations about what will happen if you create more support for yourself.

You Don't Think You Deserve It

If you have very negative, critical beliefs about yourself, you may not think that you deserve to have support from yourself or others. Unfortunately, an unsupportive and critical attitude makes achieving your healthy goals very difficult to do. Honestly ask yourself: Who deserves support and who doesn't? What disqualified you from getting support? Your conclusions about yourself and what you deserve could have a big impact on whether you get the necessary support for your healthy habits.

You Believe You Must Go It Alone

Do you see achieving your goals as something you must do on your own? Do you expect yourself to do what is necessary, without praise or encouragement from others? For some, healthy goals are just another example of work that must be done in a very cold, matter-of-fact manner. Wanting support and encouragement is viewed as unnecessary and even a sign of weakness. Some people can achieve their goals despite such beliefs, but why not have the benefit of a supportive environment?

Strategies for Staying on Track

The following strategies build on what you have learned in this chapter. As you read each one, think of specific ways in which you can use it in your daily routine.

Recognize the Value of Support

Envision the impact that support can have on reaching your goals. Be mindful of the benefits to other goals or areas of your life and how it can affect your overall happiness. Make it a part of your daily values and priorities. If you have children, remember that they will learn how to talk to themselves and get support by watching you.

Create Support Despite the Discomfort

You may notice some discomfort as you develop your supportive environment. It may come from the awkwardness of talking to yourself in a new way, or from taking the risk of asking others for help. Awkward, self-conscious, and uncomfortable feelings may be along for the ride during the early stages of creating a supportive world. Stay with it, keep practicing the solution, and don't get overly distracted by these feelings.

Create Clear Expectations

Do you have an image of how you expect to treat yourself? You may say you want to be treated with respect, kindness, and support, but often permit yourself to talk in a less than supportive voice. Create a picture of how all people should be treated and commit yourself to it. You are no different from anyone else.

Talk to Yourself as You Would a Friend

How would you talk to a friend trying to achieve similar goals? Many people are unclear about how to talk to themselves in a supportive manner, but know exactly what they would say to a friend. If you get stumped on what to say to yourself, ask what you would say to your best friend at that moment.

Expand Your Options

You may need more or different people in your life to get the support you deserve. Get creative in expanding your possibilities. Are there coworkers, neighbors, family members, or support groups that you could go to and develop supportive relationships? Supportive people are out there, but they aren't going to come knocking on your door.

Address Other Problem Areas

If you have continued difficulty staying on track with this solution, it may be due to another problem that is not being adequately addressed. Such problems may include depression, social anxiety, or anger. Be open to using outside help, such as a mental-health professional, to help you identify and resolve underlying problems.

Do You Know How to Make Good Habits a Part of Your Life?

Each chapter in this book covers an area in which many people falter in achieving their weight-loss and exercise goals. Each hidden barrier was presented with several strategies for implementation with the hope that you would find one or more of them a good fit for your unique personality and style. The big question is: How do you maintain good health habits for the long term? This chapter is devoted to helping you think through how you will maintain the positive strategies you adopted in this book over the long run, so the achievements you have made thus far will be maintained.

What Is Keeping Good Habits?

Keeping good habits for the long run involves many different things. It means that you veer off track from your goals less often than you did before. More than that, keeping new habits means that you recognize your particular vulnerabilities in achieving your goals, whether it's unrealistic game-plan strategies, difficulty handling emotions, or a hidden agenda that's tripping you up. Keeping new habits means that you possess a confident sense of vigilance and a watchful eye on when your vulnerabilities are likely to assert themselves. When you do veer off track, you treat yourself with dignity. You take responsibility, learn from mistakes if you've made them, and get right back on track with your goals. Ideally, keeping your habits for the long run means that the new lifestyle behaviors you have adopted become second nature. Your new habits are so perfectly aligned with your deeply held needs and values that the old habits, so familiar before, seem foreign and unattractive. You have made changes for the long term.

There would be no need for this book if change were immediate and lasting. If you have used the ideas in this book to reenergize yourself to achieve your weight-loss and exercise goals, then you have experienced some initial gains. You have also learned that change is most often a process with stops and starts and reconsiderations along the way. You will inevitably experience times when you don't feel like continuing on your lifestyle plan or you are caught seemingly unaware in an old, unhealthy pattern. To successfully navigate through the change process, you will need strategies for keeping your new habits for the long run.

How Are You Doing Now?

Knowing your vulnerabilities in achieving your weight-loss and exercise goals is the first step in keeping your habits for the long run. You have probably recognized some of your tendencies as you've progressed through this book. Read the following statements to find out how you're doing now with a long-range troubleshooting plan for when your healthy goals get off track. Mark the ones that apply to you.

☐ I am generally aware of when I'm veering off track from my goals.

☐ I know my particular vulnerabilities in meeting my lifestyle goals.

☐ I have a plan for troubleshooting protential problems.

☐ I accept that change is full of stops and starts.

☐ I pick myself up and go on when I fall off track.

☐ I have a problem identifying when I get off track.

☐ I am attracted by ads that promise quick change.

☐ Maintaining lifestyle change is especially hard for me.

☐ I don't have a plan for the long run.

☐ I feel discouraged about keeping up my progress.

Maintaining your successs is relevant for everyone. However, if the last five statements described you better than the first five statements, then the strategies in this chapter may be especially important for you.

How Can You Be More Successful?

It would make for a nice fantasy to believe that once you lose the weight you want or exercise for a certain length of time, then the work is done. To be successful in the long run, you'll need to continue to apply the solutions you found in this book. In addition, the following strategies should be helpful.

Keep a Realistic Picture

A realistic picture of the change process includes an accurate estimation of the weight change you want to make, the length of time before you'll see and feel changes, and the time and energy that you'll need to commit. You may want to consult your physician to learn what is realistic for you. It will also be necessary for you to recognize and be prepared to deal with slips and mistakes in your game plan. Remember the stages of change discussed in chapter 1? You may want to review these stages and recall that most people don't make lasting change on the first try.

In addition to creating realistic expectations of the change process, you should also envision the process lasting for as long as possible. Ideally, you will think of your weight-loss and exercise game plan as simply part of your lifestyle, without an ending point. Try to avoid thinking in quick, short-term time frames, as that doesn't allow enough time for new actions to become lasting habits.

Be Open to Your Vulnerability

Throughout this book you have learned that slips, mistakes, and difficulties are part of the process. Hopefully, each chapter helped you identify your particular issues that can cause problems with achieving your weight-loss and exercise goals. For you it may be a difficulty coping with negative emotions, focusing, or keeping yourself responsible to the work. Maybe you're struggling with a hidden agenda. Everyone has issues that make them vulnerable to getting off track. Having such issues isn't the problem, if they can be identified and addressed. The critical problem is when you don't know or are unwilling to confront why you're getting off track.

As part of your open and proactive attitude, you may want to create the following worksheet to help you stay on top of what gets you off track. You can type the questions on a half sheet of paper, leaving adequate space to answer each. Your answers should be brief, specific, and concrete, so that when you go back and reread them, you'll know exactly what to do. You can call the worksheet "When I Get Off Track" or any other title you like.

1. I am having difficulty sticking to my game plan because I am (*describe your off-track thoughts and actions*).

2. When I step back and look objectively at this, I believe this is happening because (*summarize what is getting you off track*).

3. To directly address this and get back on track, I will (*be very specific and concrete*).

4. To overcome why I am getting off track, I know I can count on my (*write your strengths, skills, and other relevant resources*).

Keep this worksheet handy and review it as needed. Feel free to add or change the questions as you think would be helpful. Be creative and make up your own worksheet or visual reminder for catching and dealing with the particular issues that can get you off track.

Practice Accountability

One reason why we get off track from our healthy goals is . . . because we can. No one is going to make sure you stay on track and no one will punish you if you don't. You are left to keep yourself accountable to the work of achieving your goals. Practicing accountability to your goals means that you are actively guiding the game plan and addressing any problems and concerns that arise. To stay accountable, you'll need many of the solutions described in this book, such as taking responsibility, focusing, managing emotions, and learning from mistakes.

There is no wishful thinking or magic pill that will help you stay accountable to your goals. It involves repeatedly being aware of what you want to do and then owning up to what you did do. If you followed through on your game plan, note it and provide a positive reaction or praise. If you didn't like your actions, make it your business to understand and learn from what happened. Do each often enough, and you'll begin to build a strong habit of accountability.

There are a number of tools and strategies to help you stay accountable to your game plan. You can check in with a friend who is also doing similar work, or you can participate in a support group. Putting your work on paper can also help keep you on track. Examples include writing specific goals in your daily planner and tracking your actions in an eating and exercise log. You can also create your own worksheets to help you stay accountable to what you have learned in this book. For example, you can use or adapt the following list:

1. I want to see myself doing (*very clear, detailed picture*).

2. To make this happen, I need to (*be specific*).

3. Doing this will be well worth it because (*review your motivation*).

4. After I do it, I will (*how you will respond to what you do*).

Write the list on an index card and review it as often as you think is necessary. You may want to get in the habit of rewriting it every morning or reading it before you get home.

Make Your Habits Part of a Healthy Lifestyle

While this book has focused on weight-loss and exercise goals, there are many other aspects of your life that will contribute to a healthy lifestyle. For example, other things you can do for a healthy body include: getting physical checkups as recommended for your age, taking vitamins or supplements as suggested by your physician, and reducing stress and muscle tension. Your healthy lifestyle also includes your emotional well-being. A healthy emotional lifestyle includes: working toward more effective, collaborative relationships with others, doing more meaningful activities for yourself, lowering frustration and stress, and balancing personal time with all of your other responsibilities.

The previous examples will help you create a healthier way of living, which will also directly help you stay on track with your weight-loss and exercise goals. Whenever you direct your efforts toward healthier choices, you are reinforcing your ideas about the importance and value of such pursuits. The different aspects of a healthy lifestyle also encourage or feed off one another. Rather than have your weight loss and exercise goals exist in a vacuum, place them in a context of your entire self working to become a healthier and happier person.

Make Your Habits Part of Your Self-Image

Anyone who is trying to lose weight and exercise knows that healthy habits don't initially feel easy and natural. Yet that is exactly what you want to aim for. Try to think of yourself as someone who *does* eat in healthy moderate proportions and who *does* value exercise and builds it into their schedule. Create an image of yourself as someone who successfully manages pressures, distractions, and emotions in order to stay on track with lifestyle goals. This will take time and many repetitions. Don't assume it's wrong because it feels awkward or doesn't exactly fit you now.

While you build your actions into a new way of thinking about yourself, you will also want to stop and challenge your old habits of thinking about yourself. Watch out for conclusions or labels identifying yourself as someone who can't make healthy lifestyle changes. An example is responding to a slip with "I am such an undisciplined person" or "I'm just a pretty lazy person." Such extreme conclusions reinforce your belief that you aren't the kind of person who can really be successful at making change.

Why Are You Getting off Track?

It's important to respect the challenge of keeping your habits for the long run. As part of this, continue to develop your understanding of what could get you off track in maintaining your new habits. The following areas are common reasons why people get off track with maintaining their habits.

Drifting Back to Old Habits

Drifting back to old habits is a common phenomenon for anyone trying to change and improve themselves. This is why professional athletes continue to practice their basic skills. Old habits have been around for a long time and don't just fade away nicely. Whether it is a habit of impulsively eating when bored or putting off exercise, there will be a tendency to drift back into these older habits. Don't get overly upset or surprised when this happens. Catching the drift and setting yourself back on track is part of the work of creating habits for the long run.

Not Rewarding Yourself

Although rewarding yourself has been discussed throughout this book, it deserves repeating here. New habits require reinforcement. Keep in mind that your off-track habits, such as snacking and putting off exercise, get an immediate reinforcement. Your healthy habits must compete with these old habits, and your job is to make sure they prevail. Rewarding yourself can take many forms. From a quick compliment to yourself to buying yourself new pants, you are in charge of delivering the reinforcement.

Thinking in All-or-Nothing Terms

When you think in an all-or-nothing style, everything fits into one of two categories. Either you are on top of your game or you are lazy. Either you are healthy or you are not. You are a winner or a loser. Other people are in your corner or they are against you. There is no room for complexity, understanding the change process, or any gray areas. This type of thinking can get you off track because it doesn't reflect what is actually happening. You won't catch the accurate reasons for your difficulties or what you need to learn. You will be inclined to expect too much of yourself and will have to eventually deal with painful, discouraging labels you use to describe yourself. You and your change efforts can't be summed up in one of two categories, so don't try.

Wanting the Quick Fix

There's no way to get around it: Creating new eating and exercise habits is work. While it's natural to want the work to end, some people get attached to the idea of the quick fix. The quick fix may involve very little effort, like taking pills, or doing the work for a short period of time. Either way, you're looking for an alternative to sustained, hard effort. Most people find that this usually doesn't work for any significant pursuit in life. Why should weight loss and exercise be any different?

Unresolved Problems

Throughout this book, the Why Are You Getting off Track? sections have discussed problems or issues that may need attention. Your weight-loss and exercise game plan takes place within the context of your complicated life. Sometimes other problems will overshadow or interfere with your healthy goals and make success seem impossible. Whether the problem relates to a conflict with an unsupportive partner, low self-esteem, or a lack of motivation, the problem may need more attention and treatment than you have been giving it. (See Resources for assistance.)

Strategies for Staying on Track

To enhance your ability to keep your habits for the long run, read through the following strategies and try those that you think may work for you.

Evaluate Yourself Regularly

Set aside time on a regular basis to review your goals, game-plan strategies, and troubleshooting plan. Some people will end up meeting with themselves on the same day of the month on a once-a-month basis, while others prefer to meet much more frequently. Be honest in your evaluation of your progress, review graphs you have made of your accomplishments, and plan for potential future difficulties.

Reward Yourself Liberally

The best way to help yourself repeat a behavior is to reward yourself. Rewards might include positive self-praise, a long bath with candles, or even a trip to an exotic destination. Reward yourself as soon as you notice yourself performing positive actions toward weight loss and exercise. Tell others your good news and have them comment as well.

Reread This Book

Reread the chapters in this book that are most relevant to you on a regular basis. Or, reread this chapter to review your troubleshooting plan during your regular meetings with yourself. Keep practicing the exercises to challenge some of your more persistent behaviors.

Know When to Seek Consultation

An openness to acknowledging when you need outside consultation is an important part of reaching any significant goal. While you have many personal resources to guide you to success, sometimes you will need to make changes and add to your current game plan. Whether you consult with a family member, friend, physician, or mental-health professional, there is much to be gained from the experience and perspective of others.

Never Give Up

There is hope—a lot of it—if you can muster up the strength and commitment to persevere. When you are particularly discouraged, do something that brings you some pleasure, and then get back on the horse. There are many solutions for weight loss, including behavioral strategies, medications, and surgery. And there are many solutions for exercising that you may find interesting and fun. So don't give up. With the strategies presented in this book and your long-range plan, you are well on your way to achieving your weight-loss and exercise goals.

Resources

Authors' Website

OnTrack Solutions
e-mail: www.ontracksolutions.net
For additional information, individual coaching, and consultation services

Professional Referrals

American Psychological Association Help Center
www.helping.apa.org
750 N. First Street NE
Washington, DC 20002
(800) 964-2000
Referrals and information for professional help

Nutrition, Exercise, and Health Information

Nutrition and Your Health: Dietary Guidelines for Americans, 5th Ed.
www.health.gov/dietaryguidelines
(888) 878-3256
Joint publication of the U.S. Depatrments of Health and Human Services and Agriculture

BMI Calculator:
http/nlbisupport.com/bmi/bmicalc.htm
National Heart, Lung & Blood Institute's Body Mass Index Calculator

National Academy of Sciences Report:
www.nap.edu/books/0309085373/html

American Heart Association
www.americanheart.org
National Center
7272 Greenville Avenue
Dallas, TX 75231
(800) 242-8721
Nutrition, exercise and fitness, and heart-healthy information

American Diabetes Association
www.diabetes.org
Attn: National Call Center
1701 North Beauregard
Alexandria, VA 22311
(800) 342-2383
Information about health and nutrition and diabetes

Health and Human Services (HHS)
www.healthfinder.gov
HHS gateway to reliable health information

References

Higgins, E. T. 2000. Making a good decision: Value from fit. *American Psychologist* 55:1217–1230.

Kabat-Zinn, J. 1990. *Full Catastrophe Living: Using the Wisdom of Your Body and Mind to Face Pain, Stress, and Illness.* New York: Dell Publishing.

Knowler, W. C., E. Barrett-Connor, S. E. Fowler, R. F. Hamman, J. M. Lachin, E. A. Walker, and D. M. Nathan, Diabetes Prevention Program Research Group. 2002. Reduction in the incidence of type 2 diabetes with lifestyle intervention or metformin. *New England Journal of Medicine* 346:393–403.

Leahy, R. 1999. Strategic self-limitation. *Journal of Cognitive Psychotherapy: An International Journal* 13:275–293.

Prochaska, J. O., and C. C. DiClemente. 1983. Stages and processes of self-change in smoking: Toward an integrative model of change. *Journal of Consulting and Clinical Psychology* 5:390–395.

Prochaska, J. O., J. C. Norcross, and C. C. DiClemente. 1994. *Changing for Good: A Revolutionary Six-Stage Program for Overcoming Bad Habits and Moving Your Life Positively Forward.* New York: Avon Books, Inc.

Smith, H. W. 1994. *The 10 Natural Laws of Successful Time and Life Management: Proven Strategies for Increased Productivity and Inner Peace.* New York: Warner Books, Inc.

Thayer, R. 2001. *Calm Energy: How People Regulate Mood with Food and Exercise.* New York: Oxford University Press.

U.S. Department of Agriculture and U.S. Department of Health and Human Services. 2000. *Nutrition and Your Health: Dietary Guidelines for Americans*, 5th ed. Home and Garden Bulletin No. 232.

Lynette A. Menefee, Ph.D., is a licensed psychologist and Assistant Professor of Psychiatry and Human Behavior at Jefferson Medical College in Philadelphia. Her clinical practice has focused on helping individuals overcome difficulties with behavior change as it relates to health and quality of life. She also conducts research and treats individuals with chronic pain conditions and chronic illness. She is a member of the American Psychological Association, the Society for Behavioral Medicine, and the American Pain Society. Menefee has presented and published in a variety of medical and psychological forums.

Daniel R. Somberg, Ph.D., is an assistant professor at the University of Missouri, Kansas City School of Medicine, teaching cognitive behavioral therapy to psychiatric residents. He is a licensed psychologist, working in private practice and at a community mental health center in Kansas City. Somberg's rich clinical experience and research into the latest literature on the process of change has led him to an expert's understanding of what makes for successful change and what gets in the way. Somberg has published articles in several professional journals and is a member of the American Psychological Association.

The authors can be reached at their Web site: www.ontracksolutions.net.

Some Other
New Harbinger Titles

Stop Worrying Abour Your Health, Item SWYH $14.95

The Vulvodynia Survival Guide, Item VSG $15.95

The Multifidus Back Pain Solution, Item MBPS $12.95

Move Your Body, Tone Your Mood, Item MBTM $17.95

The Chronic Illness Workbook, Item CNIW $16.95

Coping with Crohn's Disease, Item CPCD $15.95

The Woman's Book of Sleep, Item WBS $14.95

The Trigger Point Therapy Workbook, Item TPTW $19.95

Fibromyalgia and Chronic Myofascial Pain Syndrome, second edition, Item FMS2 $19.95

Kill the Craving, Item KC $18.95

Rosacea, Item ROSA $13.95

Thinking Pregnant, Item TKPG $13.95

Shy Bladder Syndrome, Item SBDS $13.95

Help for Hairpullers, Item HFHP $13.95

Coping with Chronic Fatigue Syndrome, Item CFS $13.95

The Stop Smoking Workbook, Item SMOK $17.95

Multiple Chemical Sensitivity, Item MCS $16.95

Breaking the Bonds of Irritable Bowel Syndrome, Item IBS $14.95

Parkinson's Disease and the Art of Moving, Item PARK $16.95

The Addiction Workbook, Item AWB $18.95

The Interstitial Cystitis Survival Guide, Item ICS $15.95

Illness and the Art of Creative Self-Expression, Item EXPR $13.95

Don't Leave it to Chance, Item GMBL $13.95

Call **toll free, 1-800-748-6273,** or log on to our online bookstore at **www.newharbinger.com** to order. Have your Visa or Mastercard number ready. Or send a check for the titles you want to New Harbinger Publications, Inc., 5674 Shattuck Ave., Oakland, CA 94609. Include $4.50 for the first book and 75¢ for each additional book, to cover shipping and handling. (California residents please include appropriate sales tax.) Allow two to five weeks for delivery.

Prices subject to change without notice.